Bob

for the well-remembered
bus-stop in Kansas City –
and the Peppercorn duck club
and the (innumerable?) meetings
and Five Island

I look forward to your continued
inspiration
and
future
authorship

(enjoy the "long plane ride to Colorado Springs")
and thank you for the continuing support

Kathy Reed

FETAL ECHOCARDIOGRAPHY
An Atlas

FETAL ECHOCARDIOGRAPHY
An Atlas

Kathryn L. Reed, M.D.
Caroline F. Anderson, R.D.M.S.
Lewis Shenker, M.D.
Department of Obstetrics and Gynecology
University of Arizona
Tucson, Arizona

Illustrated by

Fred Anderson, M.F.A., Medical Illustrator

With a Contribution on Color Flow Mapping by
David J. Sahn, M.D.
Department of Pediatrics (Cardiology)
University of California at San Diego

Alan R. Liss, Inc., New York

Address all Inquiries to the Publisher
Alan R. Liss, Inc., 41 East 11th Street, New York, NY 10003

Copyright © 1988 Alan R. Liss, Inc.

All rights reserved. This book is protected by copyright. No part of it, except brief excerpts for review, may be reproduced, stored in a retrieval system, or transmitted in any form or by any means, electronic, mechanical, photocopying, recording, or otherwise, without written permission from the publisher.

Printed in the United States of America.

While the authors, editors, and publisher believe that drug selection and dosage and the specifications and usage of equipment and devices, as set forth in this book, are in accord with current recommendations and practice at the time of publication, they accept no legal responsibility for any errors or omissions, and make no warranty, express or implied, with respect to material contained herein. In view of ongoing research, equipment modifications, changes in governmental regulations and the constant flow of information relating to drug therapy, drug reactions and the use of equipment and devices, the reader is urged to review and evaluate the information provided in the package insert or instructions for each drug, piece of equipment or device for, among other things, any changes in the instructions or indications of dosage or usage and for added warnings and precautions.

Library of Congress Cataloging-in-Publication Data

Reed, Kathryn L.
    Fetal echocardiography.
    Includes index.
    1. Echocardiography—Atlases. 2. Fetal heart—
Imaging—Atlases. I. Anderson, C.F. (Caroline Frances)
II. Shenker, Lewis. III. Title. [DNLM: 1. Echo-
cardiography—atlases. 2. Fetal Heart—abnormalities—
atlases. 3. Fetal Heart—anatomy—atlases. 4. Prenatal
Diagnosis—atlases.   WQ 17 R324f]
RG628.3E34R44 1988   618.92′107543   88-686
ISBN 0-8451-4250-X

CONTENTS

	Preface	vii
1	Introduction	1
2	Fetal Heart: Anatomy and Physiology	5
3	Methods of Examination: Two-Dimensional	11
4	The Abnormal Fetal Heart	47
5	M-Mode Echocardiography	103
6	Doppler Echocardiography	109
7	Fetal Cardiac Arrhythmias	115
8	Color Flow Mapping By David J. Sahn	125
	Index	135

PREFACE

Fetal echocardiography has evolved as an independent discipline since 1970. Resolution capabilities of two-dimensional equipment have improved markedly during this span of time. The use of M-mode echocardiography has allowed identification of fetal arrhythmias and improved quantitation of the sizes of fetal cardiac structures. Finally, the introduction of Doppler ultrasound to the study of fetuses has enabled a better understanding of both normal and abnormal cardiovascular physiology.

This atlas is a basic guide to examinations of the fetal heart. It is intended for use by everyone concerned with fetal cardiac ultrasound, including those in the fields of obstetrics, pediatrics, cardiology, imaging, physiology, anatomy, and genetics.

The field is in evolution, and improved technology and imaging skills will add information beyond what is in this guide. However, we hope that this work will be used to orient the beginner and that it will provide a service to those who continue the study of the fetal cardiovascular system.

Many hands, eyes, and minds have cooperated to generate this book. Dr. Sahn and Dr. Shenker originally conspired with Dr. Reed and Sarah Scagnelli, R.D.M.S., to systematically study the cardiovascular system of the fetus with Doppler ultrasound. The idea was thus introduced that the fetal heart was accessible to ultrasound examination. Susie (Caroline F.) Anderson has been performing ultrasound studies since 1973, with a special interest in the fetus. The combination of technician, obstetrician, and pediatric cardiologist proved propitious and a vigorous study of the fetal heart and cardiovascular system commenced in 1980. None of this would have been possible without the support of other colleagues. We especially thank Drs. Marx, Allen, and Donnerstein, pediatric cardiologists, who have suffered with us in understanding the cardiovascular anatomy and physiology of the fetus; Dr. Steven Goldman, a cardiologist who has generously shared his interest in physiology; Nydia Borjon, R.D.M.S., who with her constant support has allowed us the time to create this work; and C.D. Christian, M.D., Ph.D., chairman of the Department of Obstetrics and Gynecology at the University of Arizona, who allowed the group to seek its highest level of cooperation.

Kathryn L. Reed, M.D.
Caroline F. Anderson, R.D.M.S.
Lewis Shenker, M.D.

1

Introduction

With the use of high-resolution equipment, the fetal heart can be visualized in nearly every ultrasound examination. Populations that should be offered careful examinations of the fetal heart are listed in Table 1–1 [1]. They include those with a positive family history of problems with congenital cardiac anomalies. There are reports of a 3–4% incidence of congenital cardiac disease in this group. There is a potential of up to 50% recurrence of cardiac disease in genetic conditions such as Marfan's syndrome. Certain maternal conditions predispose the fetus to the development of cardiac disease. Women with insulin-dependent diabetes have a 3–4-fold increase in fetal anomalies, and one-third of these are cardiac. Gestational diabetics, or any diabetic at risk for a macrosomic infant, can have fetuses with enlarged hearts and thickened ventricles. Women with connective tissue

TABLE 1-1. Fetal Cardiac Evaluation: High-Risk Groups

History of congenital heart disease	***Abnormal pregnancy***
Self	Known or suspected fetal
Child	anomaly based on:
Relative	Ultrasound
Predisposing maternal conditions	Amniotic fluid volume
Diabetes	Fetal growth
Insulin-dependent	Chromosomes
Gestational	Multiple gestation
Connective tissue disease	Persistent malpresentation
Isoimmunization	Fetal cardiac arrhythmia
Phenylketonuria	
Advanced maternal age	
Exposure to teratogens/drugs	
Phenytoin	
Lithium	
Alcohol	
Isotretinoin	
Oral contraceptives	
Rubella	
Antihypertensives	
Tocolytics	

disease, especially those with anti-Ro antibody, may have fetuses with complete heart block and possibly anatomic anomalies. If isoimmunization complicates the pregnancy, the fetus may develop hemolytic anemia and congestive heart failure. Women with phenylketonuria, whose diets are not controlled, may have fetuses with congenital heart defects. Women aged 35 or older have an increased risk of delivering a child with a chromosome anomaly, which may be complicated by a cardiac defect.

Exposure to teratogens or other drugs that potentially alter fetal cardiac function comprise another group. Phenytoin is reported to increase congenital defects, including cardiac defects. Lithium is reported to contribute to the incidence of Ebstein's anomaly, among other congenital defects that may be cardiac. Alcohol is another potential source of fetal cardiac abnormalities. Isotretinoin is a potent teratogen, and septal defects have been reported with its use. Oral contraceptives are a possible source of fetal cardiac defects. Exposure to the rubella virus has been reported to cause pulmonic stenosis. Antihypertensive agents are likely to alter the cardiac function of the fetus. Tocolytic agents may change fetal cardiac function, including heart rate. Indomethacin has been reported to decrease the size of the ductus arteriosus.

Another group of potentially abnormal fetuses is ascertained as the pregnancy progresses. These include pregnancies with abnormalities detectable by ultrasound or karyotyping, increased amniotic fluid volume (associated with chromosome or other anomalies), and decreased amniotic fluid volume (associated with intrauterine growth retardation or renal anomalies). Intrauterine growth retardation may be associated with fetal anomalies; macrosomia may be associated with maternal diabetes. The presence of hydrops may indicate that a fetal cardiac arrhythmia is present or that a cardiac anomaly has resulted in the development of congestive heart failure. Arrhythmias should be investigated with fetal cardiac ultrasound examinations. Tachyarrhythmias may result in fetal hydrops, and bradyarrhythmias also may be complicated by cardiac anomalies and failure.

TABLE 1-2. Lesions Difficult or Impossible to Exclude With Fetal Echocardiography

Patent foramen ovale
Patent ductus arteriosus
Small septal defect
Minor valvular anomalies
Pulmonary venous abnormalities

TABLE 1-3. Karyotypic Abnormalities That May Lead to Cardiac Abnormalities

Trisomy	%	PDA	Septal defects	Other anomalies
21	50	X	X	AV canal, T of F
18	50	X	X	Bicuspid AO, PA
13	80	X	X	Dextrocardia

PDA = patent ductus arteriosus; AV = atrioventricular; T of F = tetralogy of Fallot; AO = aorta; PA = pulmonary artery.

The timing of fetal echocardiographic studies will vary with the reason for the examination. When a history of previous problems is present, or the suspicion of a congenital cardiac lesion is present, the study can be performed at 16–18 weeks. For purposes of confirmation, or a more complete examination, the study can be repeated at 24–28 weeks. If an indication arises during the pregnancy, the examination can be performed at any time. Third-trimester examinations can vary in difficulty with the position of the fetus.

Various cardiac lesions are difficult or impossible to detect in the human fetus with the use of ultrasound (Table 1–2). Some of these difficulties rest with the fact that the foramen ovale and ductus arteriosus are normally patent in the fetus. Premature closure of these structures, in fact, can result in fetal morbidity. Atrial septal defects can be detected if they are sufficiently large. Ventricular septal defects can be difficult or almost impossible to detect. Valvular abnormalities may not be detected or may become more obvious after birth as the ventricular pressures and volumes change. Abnormalities of pulmonary venous return may be difficult to detect, given the size and normal intrauterine volume flow in the fetus.

IMPORTANT POINTS

If a cardiac anomaly is present, a karyotypic abnormality may be present (12–35%) [2].

If a karyotypic abnormality is present, a cardiac anomaly may be present (50–80%) (Table 1–3) [1].

If fetal anatomy (excluding the heart) is abnormal, there is a 26% chance that the heart is also abnormal [3].

Obstruction of fetal cardiac blood flow can result in fluid collections easily identified in the fetus; an example of this is right atrial enlargement in the presence of pulmonic stenosis and absent ventricular septal defect.

Tricuspid insufficiency is associated with increased fetal morbidity, especially if associated with a cardiac anomaly [4].

The spectrum of cardiac disease detected in the fetus is different from that detected in the stillborn or the newborn [5].

Complete heart block may indicate the presence of anti-Ro antibody [6]. If no anti-Ro antibody is found in association with congenital heart block in the fetus, a careful examination of the fetal heart is indicated for the presence of other cardiac anomalies [7].

Detection of fetal cardiac anomalies can result in better care for the fetus:

    Proper selection of time, location, and personnel for the delivery

    Preparation of the parents

        obstetricians

        neonatologists

        pediatric cardiologists

The best work comes from a cooperative effort:

    Obstetrician/perinatologist

    Pediatrician/neonatologist

    Pediatric cardiologist

    Radiologist/technologist

REFERENCES

1. Reed KL, Sahn DJ: A proposal for referral patterns for fetal cardiac studies. Semin Ultrasound 5:249–252, 1984.
2. Copel JA, Cullen M, Green J, et al: Congenital heart disease diagnosed by fetal echocardiography and chromosomal abnormalities. Meeting of the Society of Perinatal Obstetricians, Lake Buena Vista, FL, February 5–6, 1987 (abstr).
3. Copel JA, Pilu G, Kleinman CS: Congenital heart disease and extracardiac anomalies: Associations and indications for fetal echocardiography. Am J Obstet Gynecol 154:1121–1132, 1986.
4. Silverman NH, Kleinman CS, Rudolph AM, et al: Fetal atrioventricular valve insufficiency associated with nonimmune hydrops: A two-dimensional echocardiographic and pulsed Doppler study. Circulation 72:825–832, 1985.
5. Allan LD, Crawford DC, Anderson RH, Tynan M: Spectrum of congenital heart disease detected echocardiographically in prenatal life. Br Heart J 54:523–526, 1985.
6. Litsey SE, Noonan JA, O'Conner WN, et al: Maternal connective tissue disease and congenital heart block. N Engl J Med 312:98–100, 1985.
7. Shenker L, Reed KL, Anderson CF, et al: Congenital heart block and cardiac anomalies in the absence of maternal connective tissue disease. Am J Obstet Gynecol 157:248–253, 1987.

2

Fetal Heart: Anatomy and Physiology

An examination of the human fetal heart requires an understanding of the differences between the fetal heart and the adult heart. Most previous studies of the fetal heart were performed in animals, with obvious differences from human hearts. The adult human heart has been studied in some detail, due to the larger size and greater accessibility.

The human fetal heart has been examined recently with ultrasound techniques and with fetal electronic monitoring. With both methods, anatomical and physiological properties can be described.

ANATOMY

The foramen ovale is patent in the fetus, allowing blood to flow from the right atrium into the left atrium (Fig. 2-1, Table 2-1). The ductus arteriosus is also normally patent; it provides a substantial channel through which the blood flows from the right ventricle to the descending aorta. After delivery the ductus arteriosus normally closes and is present as a ligamentous structure later in life.

The shape of the fetal ventricles is more round than that of the adult ventricles. The right and left ventricles are hemispherical in cross section in the fetus. After birth the right ventricle gradually assumes a crescentic shape, while the left ventricle hypertrophies physiologically and becomes more circular (Fig. 2-2) [1].

The thickness of the ventricular walls and the intraventricular septum are approximately equal in the fetus [2]. This differs from the adult heart, in which the left ventricular free wall is larger than the right ventricular free wall (Fig. 2-2).

The shape of the fetal ventricles are more similar in cross section than in the adult heart (Fig. 2-2). The fetal right ventricle is similar in size [3] or slightly larger in diameter [4] than the left ventricle. The volume of the right ventricle appears to be larger than the volume of the left ventricle, due not only to differences in diameters, but to the position of the right ventricular outflow tract. The right ventricular outflow tract is more superior and anterior than the left ventricular outflow tract.

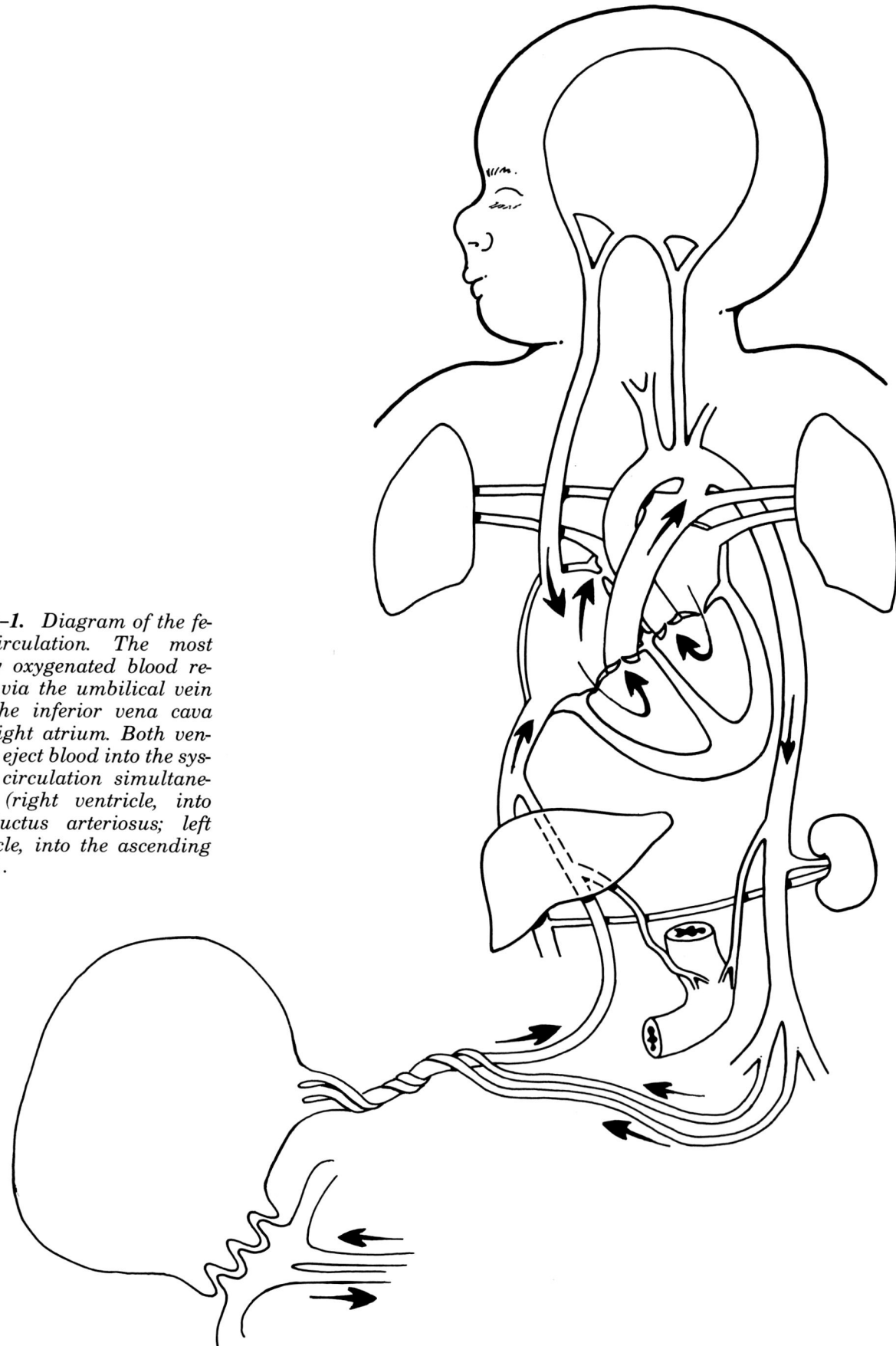

Fig. 2-1. Diagram of the fetal circulation. The most highly oxygenated blood returns via the umbilical vein into the inferior vena cava and right atrium. Both ventricles eject blood into the systemic circulation simultaneously (right ventricle, into the ductus arteriosus; left ventricle, into the ascending aorta).

TABLE 2-1. Fetal Cardiac Anatomy

Patent foramen ovale
Patent ductus arteriosus
Round ventricles
Right ventricle larger than left

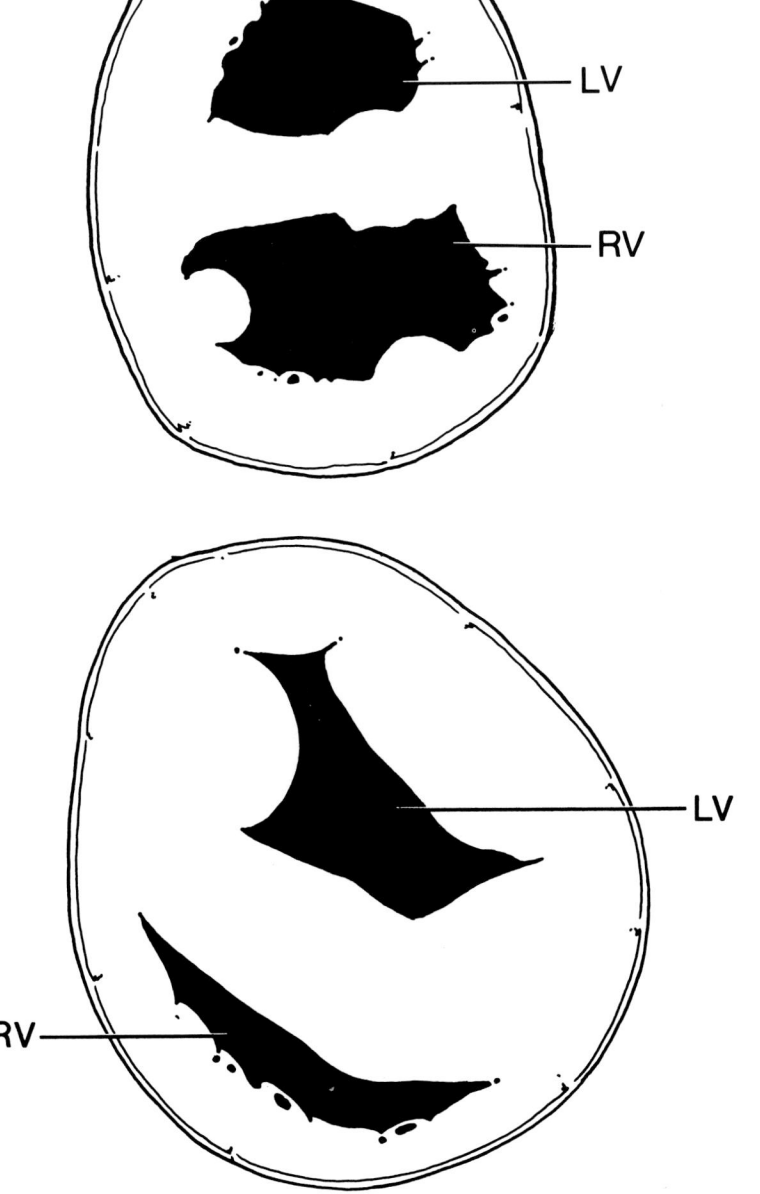

Fig. 2-2. Diagrammatic cross section of the fetal heart (**a**) at birth and (**b**) after normal serial circulation has been established. Note the relative similarity in cross-sectional appearance immediately after birth and the physiological hypertrophy of the left ventricle (LV) later in life. RV = right ventricle. (Adapted from Versprille et al., 1978, with permission of the publisher.)

PHYSIOLOGY

In the human fetus, the organ of oxygenation is the placenta, rather than the lungs. Patterns of intracardiac blood flow in the fetus differ from those present after birth, since the lungs are primarily bypassed.

Both fetal ventricles eject blood into the systemic circulation simultaneously (Table 2-2). The right ventricle ejects into the main pulmonary artery, the ductus arteriosus, and the descending aorta. In the fetal lamb, 7–8% of the combined ventricular output (combination of the right and left ventricular outputs) passes through the lungs and into the left atrium [5]. The left ventricle ejects blood into the ascending aorta and its branches (the brachiocephalic trunk, left common carotid artery, and left subclavian artery) and eventually into the descending aorta. Also unique to the fetus is the presence of the placental circulation, in which vascular resistance is low. The umbilical arteries are branches of the hypogastric arteries. Therefore the resistance in the descending aorta is a combination of placental resistance and peripheral vascular resistance in the lower portions of the fetus.

The right ventricle ejects more blood per beat than does the left ventricle. In the sheep the ratio of right-to-left blood flow is 60:40–65:35 [5]; in the human, by Doppler ultrasound studies, the ratio appears to be 55:45 [6–8]. The difference between the human and sheep can be attributed to the fact that the human brain, which is supplied by the left ventricle, is larger than the sheep brain.

The fetal heart rate is normally between 120 and 160 bpm. The reason for the rapidity of the fetal heart rate is unknown. Increases in heart rate to compensate for cardiovascular abnormalities are not common in the fetus. Neither fetal anemia nor chronic hypoxia are necessarily manifested by tachycardia in the fetus. The fact that the fetus does not respond with increases in heart rate may be due to decreased compliance and the size of the ventricles. After birth, heart rate gradually decreases over the first few months and year of life. Fetal blood pressure is about 65/35 mm Hg [9]. Blood pressure in the newborn infant increases to 70/50 mm Hg [9]. Prior to birth, pressures appear to be similar in both the right and left ventricles. There may be some differences based on the tapering of the ductus arteriosus and the presence of the placenta [5].

Saturation and partial pressures of oxygen in the fetus are low, by adult standards. Highest oxygen levels are present in the umbilical vein blood

TABLE 2-2. Fetal Cardiac Physiology

Parallel ventricular flow
  Right greater than left
  7–8% of total through lungs (fetal lambs)
Heart rate 120–160 bpm
Blood pressure 65/35 mm hg

	Umbilical artery	Umbilical vein
pO_2 (mm Hg)	20–22	30–35
O_2 saturation	46–51%	85%

Compliance is decreased
Hemoglobin F
Hemoglobin 16 g/dl

that flows from the placenta. This blood enters the ductus venosus and inferior vena cava. Most of this blood moves preferentially across the right atrium and foramen ovale into the left atrium, left ventricle, and ascending aorta and brain. Less-oxygenated blood in the superior vena cava, along with some blood from the inferior vena cava, flows into the right ventricle and through the ductus into the descending aorta. Because fetal blood is oxygenated via the maternal circulation, primarily at the venous level, pO_2 and saturation will mimic that of the maternal venous circulation and decrease as it passes through the fetus. The fetal arterial circulation has even lower levels of pO_2 and oxygen saturation. Data from umbilical artery samplings have preliminarily shown that the pH is 7.27–7.45 and pO_2 is 35 mm Hg [10].

The compliance of the fetal heart is lower than in the infant and the adult. Animal studies in sheep hearts have shown that pressure-volume loops are shifted to the left in the fetus [11]. Doppler ultrasound studies performed from 16 to 42 weeks gestation have shown results that confirm that the human fetal heart is less compliant than the adult heart [12].

The fetal hemoglobin (16 g/dl) is higher than in the infant or the adult, and the fetal hemoglobin (F) has a greater affinity to oxygen than does adult hemoglobin (A).

At birth, several changes take place. Placental blood flow ceases, and the lungs become the means of oxygenation. With the onset of breathing of air, pulmonary vascular resistance decreases, pulmonary blood flow increases, and left atrial and left ventricular pressures increase relative to right atrial and right ventricular pressures. The arterial pO_2 increases to 80–90 mm Hg. The foramen ovale closes, as does the ductus arteriosus. Several of these changes have been studied using Doppler echocardiography [13].

Thus the human fetal heart differs in multiple ways from the cardiovascular anatomy and physiology as it is understood in the adult. It is important to keep these differences in mind, not only to improve the accurate assessment of the normal human fetus, but to further understand, predict and possibly prevent the development of fetal compromise.

REFERENCES

1. Versprille A, Jansen JRC, Harinck E, et al: Functional interaction of both ventricles at birth and the changes during the neonatal period in relation to the change of geometry. In Longo LD, Reneau DD (eds): Fetal and Newborn Cardiovascular Physiology, Vol. 1. New York: Garland, 1978, pp 399–413.
2. St. John Sutton MG, Raichlen JS, Reichek N, Huff DS: Quantitative assessment of right and left ventricular growth in the human fetal heart: A pathoanatomic study. Circulation 70:935–941, 1984.
3. DeVore GR, Siassi B, Platt LD: Fetal echocardiography, IV. M-mode assessment of ventricular size and contractility during the second and third trimesters of pregnancy in the normal fetus. Am J Obstet Gynecol 150:981–988, 1984.
4. Silverman NH, Golbus MS: Echocardiographic techniques for assessing normal and abnormal fetal cardiac anatomy. J Am Coll Cardiol 5:20S–29S, 1985.
5. Rudolph AR: Distribution and regulation of blood flow in the fetal and neonatal lamb. Circ Res 57:811–821, 1985.
6. Reed KL, Meijboom EJ, Scagnelli SA, et al: Cardiac Doppler flow velocities in human fetuses. Circulation 73:41–46, 1986.

7. Kenny JF, Plappert T, Doubilet et al: Changes in intracardiac blood flow velocities and right and left ventricular stroke volumes with gestational age in the normal human fetus: A prospective Doppler echocardiographic study. Circulation 74:1208–1216, 1986.
8. Allan LD, Chita SK, Al-Ghazali W, et al: Doppler echocardiographic evaluation of the normal heart fetal heart. Br Heart J 57:528–533, 1987.
9. Rudolph AM: Fetal circulation and cardiovascular adjustments after birth. In Rudolph AM (ed): Pediatrics, Ed. 17. New York: Appleton-Century-Crofts, 1982.
10. Nicolaides KH, Bradley RJ, Campbell S, et al: Maternal oxygen therapy for intrauterine growth retardation. Lancet 1:942–946, 1987.
11. Romero T, Covell J, Friedman WF: A comparison of pressure–volume relations of the fetal, newborn and adult heart. Am J Physiol 222:1285–1290, 1972.
12. Reed KL, Sahn DJ, Scagnelli SA, et al: Doppler echocardiographic studies of diastolic function in the human fetal heart: Changes during gestation. J Am Coll Cardiol 8:391–395, 1986.
13. Wilson N, Reed KL, Allen HD, et al: Doppler echocardiographic observations of pulmonary and transvalvular velocity changes after birth and during the early neonatal period. Am Heart J 113:750–758, 1987.

3

Methods of Examination: Two-Dimensional

Studies of the fetal heart with ultrasound are possible because the heart is a fluid-filled structure in a fetus, and the fetus is normally contained in an amniotic (fluid-filled) environment. The views of the heart are unobstructed by air in the lungs and relatively unobstructed by ribs and other fetal parts until late in gestation.

To understand the views of the fetal heart that are described and the almost limitless number that can be obtained, it is necessary to realize that there are two three-dimensional arrangements to keep in mind. 1) The fetal position inside the uterus must be determined. We locate the fetal body, head, and spine relative to the mother, so that the appropriate approaches to the fetal heart are apparent. 2) After the fetus has been otherwise studied, we concentrate on the orientation of the fetal heart within the fetal body. Initial studies of the fetal heart may be greatly assisted by having a model of the fetal heart available to orient to the position of the fetal heart being studied.

Illustrations are shown utilizing a linear-array transducer for the purpose of simplicity. For anatomical studies, we prefer the use of sector transducers due to the ease of manipulation.

The fetal heart can be evaluated from many transducer positions, limited only by rib and spine acoustical shadowing. In this book we have included the views that give the greatest amount of information and that are the most reproducible.

The fetal heart lies almost transversely in the fetal chest, in part because the fetal lungs have not yet fully expanded. The heart lies superior to the liver and stomach. Care must be taken to determine the fetal position regardless of stomach, liver, and heart positions because dextrocardia, situs inversus, and other anomalies can affect anatomical positions of these structures.

The apex of the heart lies against the left anterior chest wall, with the right ventricle most anterior and the left ventricle closest to the spine. The atria are located slightly more cephalad than the ventricles.

These ultrasound studies are oriented with the image right as the mother's right in the transverse images, and the image right toward the mother's feet in the sagittal images. In most of the cases shown, the fetus is in a cephalic presentation.

FOUR-CHAMBER VIEW

From the Apex

The fetus is lying with the left anterior chest wall toward the transducer, with the fetal spine at the 4 o'clock position, the fetal back to the maternal right, and the fetus in a cephalic presentation. This is a transverse cross-section through the fetal chest with a slight cephalad (fetal) tilt of the transducer (Fig. 3–1).

All four chambers, ventricular and atrial septae, foramen ovale and flap, tricuspid and mitral valves, and the pulmonary veins are easily visualized in this view. Although no single view can be used to rule out all cardiac defects, this is the view most easily obtained and most useful in the evaluation of the ventricular and atrial septae, chamber and valve sizes, and positions (Tables 3–1 and 3–2).

TABLE 3–1. Basic Anatomy: Four-Chamber

Ventricles appear approximately equal in size
Atria appear approximately equal in size
Left ventricle is usually closest to spine
Tricuspid valve inserts lower on septum
Foramen ovale flap is in left atrium
Pulmonary veins enter left atrium
Septae and atrioventricular valves meet in center of heart
Heart occupies approximately one-third of chest

TABLE 3–2. Fetal Cardiac Anatomy: Four-Chamber

Structures seen

Right and left ventricles	Intra-atrial septum
Right and left atria	Foramen ovale
Mitral and tricuspid valves	Pericardium
Intraventricular septum	Ventricular walls

Measurements
Compare ventricular sizes
Ventricular wall and septal thickness

Anomalies ruled out

Hypoplasia of RV or LV	Valve atresia/stenosis/insufficiency
Single ventricle	Ebstein's anomaly
Large ASD or VSD	Pericardial effusion
Atrioventricular canal defect	Dextrocardia
Double outlet right ventricle	Cardiac hypertrophy
Tetralogy of Fallot	Cardiomyopathy
Coarctation of the aorta	Situs inversus
Premature closure of the foramen	Ectopia cordis
Premature closure of the ductus	Cardiac tumors

RV = right ventricle; LV = left ventricle; ASD = atrial septal defect; VSD = ventricular septal defect.

From the Base

In the diagram (Fig. 3-2a,b), the fetus is in a cephalic presentation, with the fetal spine toward the mother's left side and the fetal right posterior chest wall toward the transducer. The ultrasound beam enters the fetal chest inferior to the scapula and transects the fetal chest with a caudal tilt to the transducer. The fetal spine is between the 10 o'clock and 11 o'clock positions. In the ultrasound and drawing (Fig. 3-2c,d), the fetus is in a breech position with the spine at the 2 o'clock position. Therefore, the right-sided fetal cardiac structures are seen to the maternal (and page) left.

In this view both atria, atrial septum, foramen ovale, pulmonary veins, tricuspid and mitral valves, ventricular septum, and ventricular chambers are seen.

FIVE-CHAMBER VIEW

This view is a slight variation of the apical four-chamber view and can be obtained by a slight fetocephalic tilt of the transducer from the plane of the apical view. The ascending aorta makes a "fifth chamber", separating the right and left atria (Fig. 3-3). The ventricular septum makes a smooth transition into the right wall of the ascending aorta. The aortic valve is also apparent.

RIGHT VENTRICULAR OUTFLOW TRACT

By moving the transducer slightly more cephalad from the five-chamber view, the right ventricular outflow tract, pulmonary artery and valve, and the ductus arteriosus can be seen exiting the superior aspect of the right ventricle, crossing to the left and entering the descending aorta (Fig. 3-4). A small portion of the transverse aortic arch can also be seen at times (depending upon transducer angulation) to the right of the pulmonary artery and ductus arteriosus.

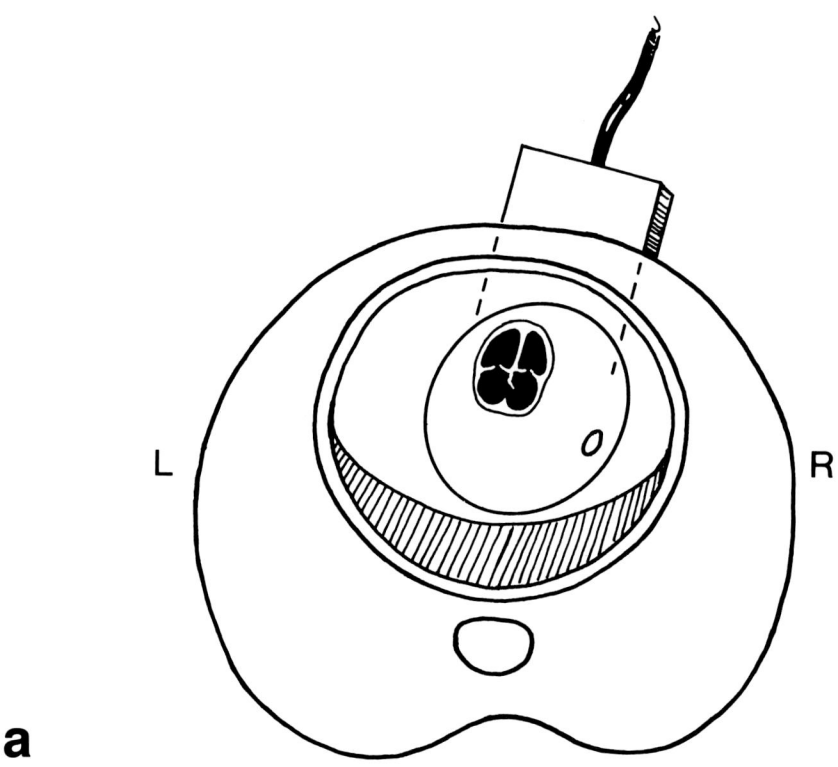

Fig. 3-1a-d. Four-chamber view from the apex. The fetus is in a cephalic presentation with the fetal spine at the 4 o'clock position. The transducer is tilted toward the fetal head. The maternal right is image right. This is the single most useful view and the easiest to reproduce. All four chambers, ventricular and atrial septae, foramen ovale and flap, and both atrioventricular valves are seen. RV = right ventricle; LV = left ventricle; RA = right atrium; LA = left atrium; FO = foramen ovale; PVn, PV = pulmonary vein; TV = tricuspid valve; MV = mitral valve; SVC = superior vena cava.

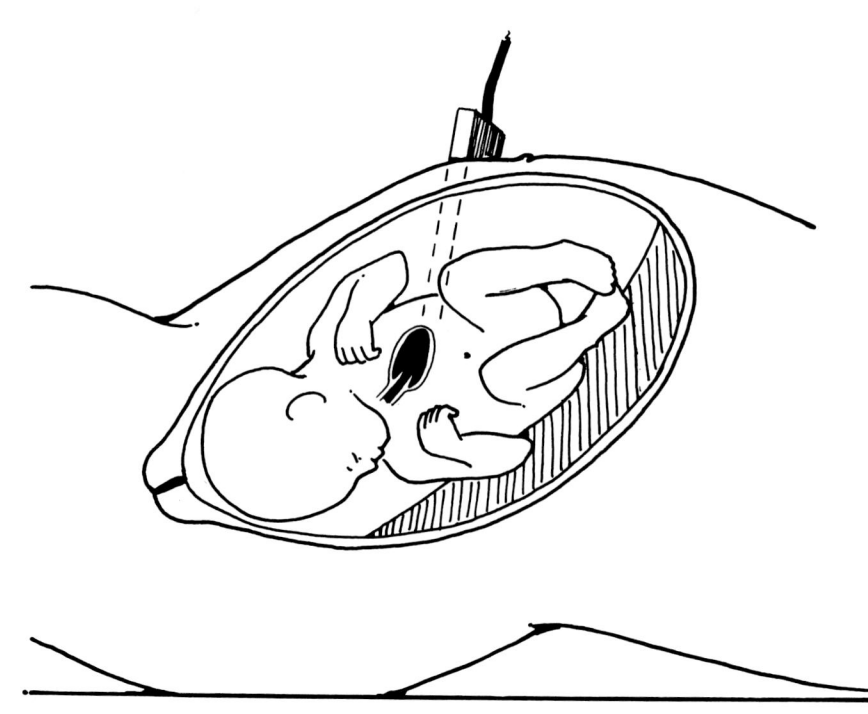

METHODS OF EXAMINATION: TWO-DIMENSIONAL

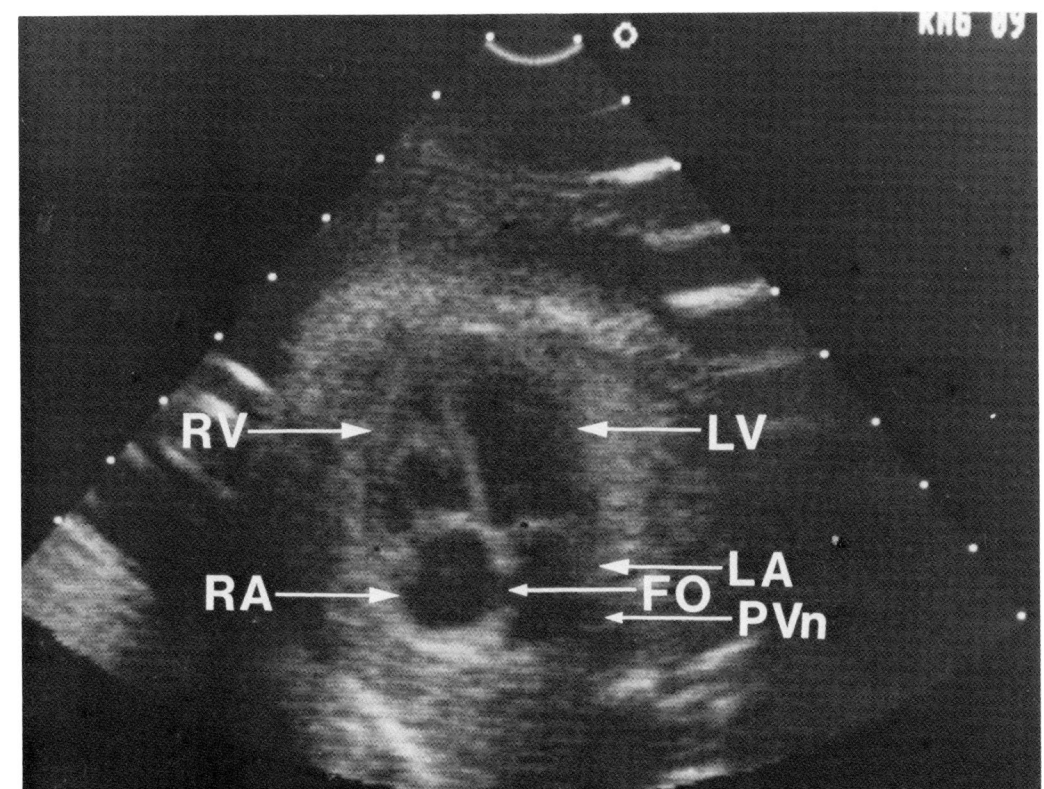

c

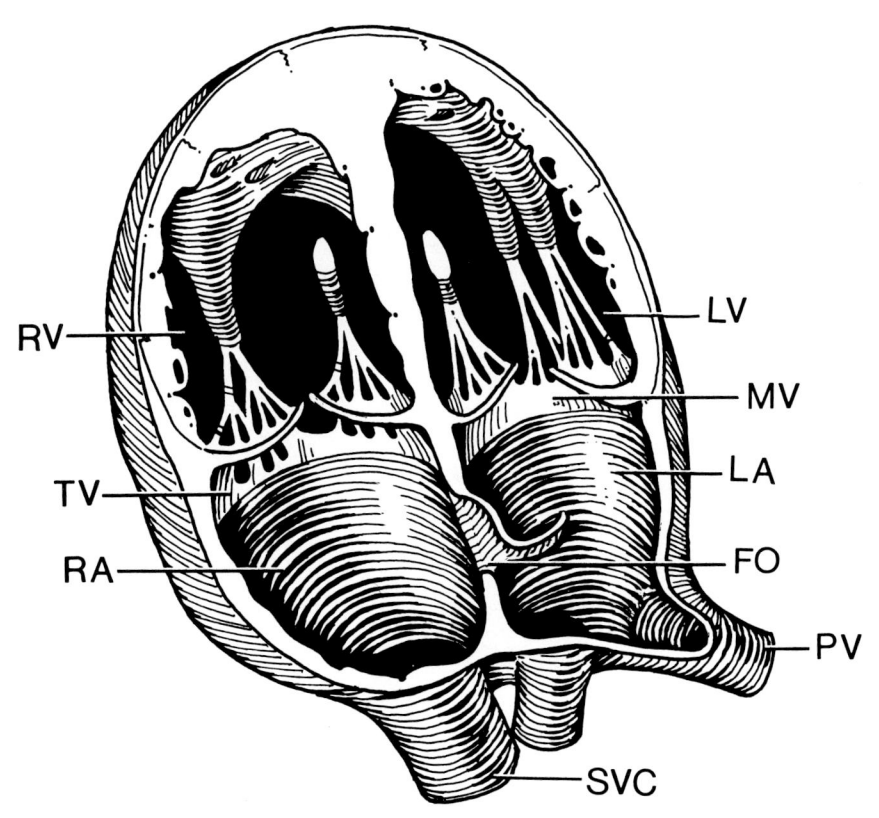

d

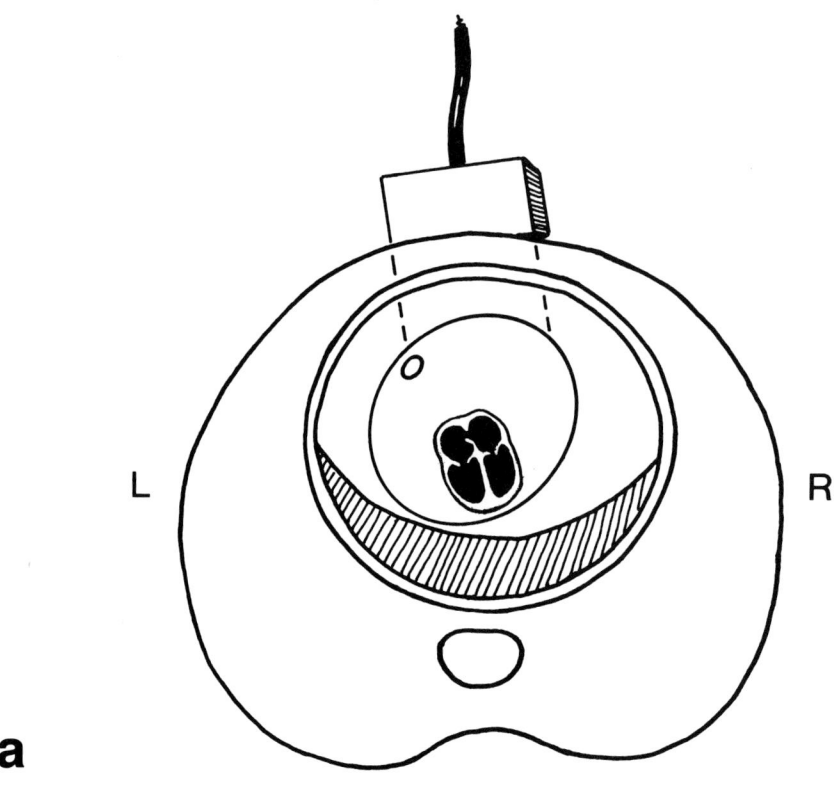

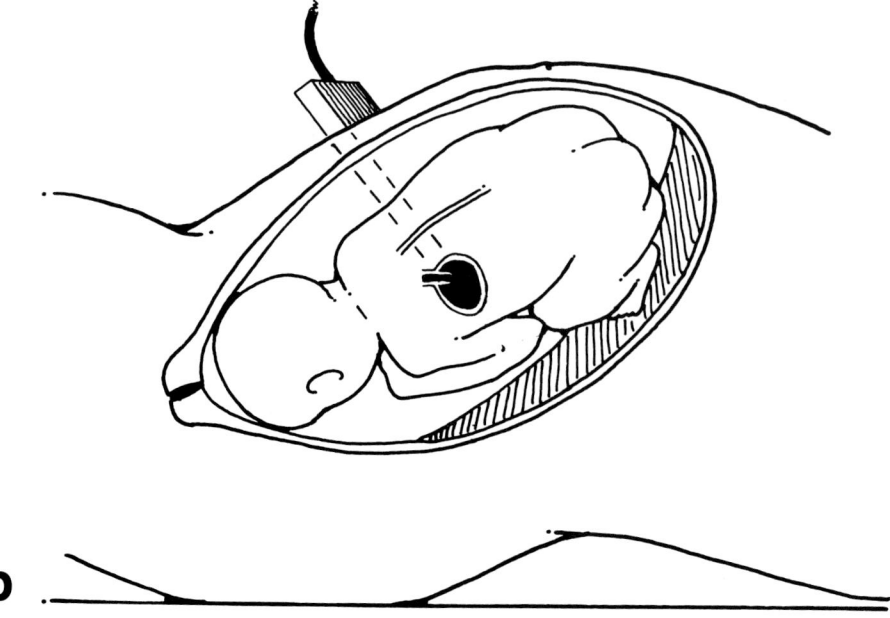

Fig. 3–2a–d. Four-chamber view from the base. **a,b:** The fetus is shown in a cephalic presentation with the spine at the 10 o'clock position, which gives a reverse view of the ultrasound image. **c,d:** The fetus is in a breech position with the spine at the 2 o'clock position. In this view, the transducer is tilted caudally from the upper posterior thorax. RV = right ventricle; LV = left ventricle; RA = right atrium; LA = left atrium; FO = foramen ovale; PVn = pulmonary vein; MV = mitral valve; TV = tricuspid valve; SV = superior vena cava.

METHODS OF EXAMINATION: TWO-DIMENSIONAL

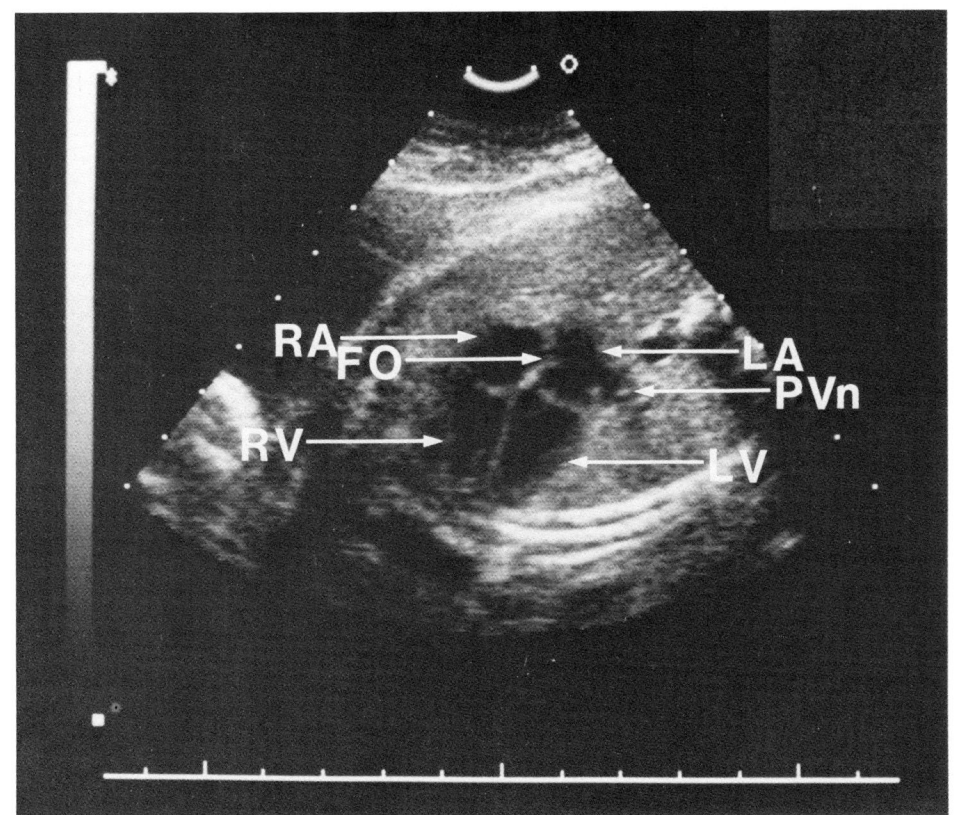

c

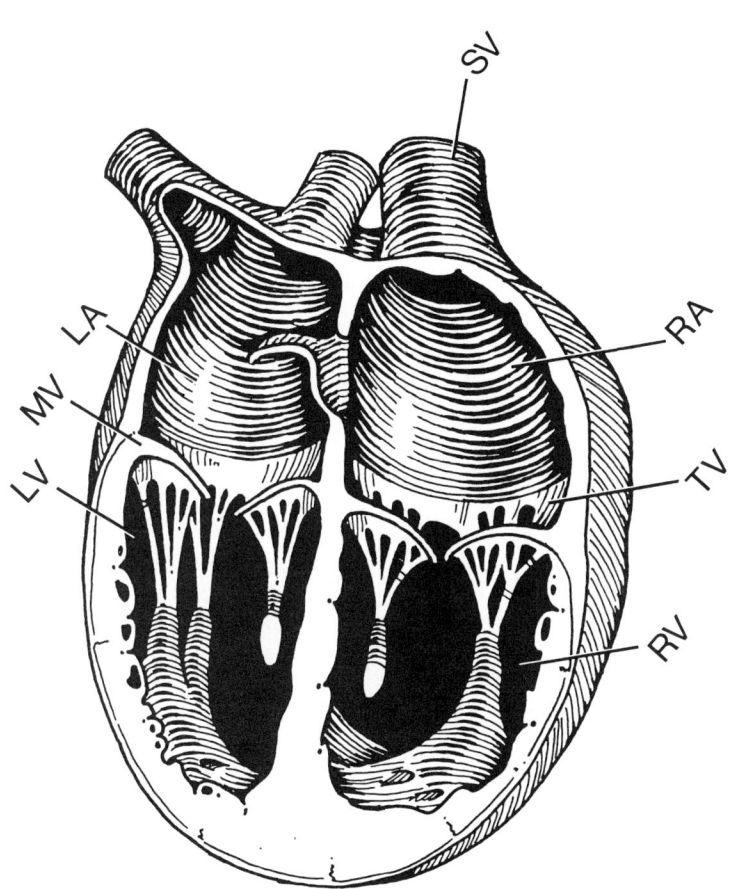

d

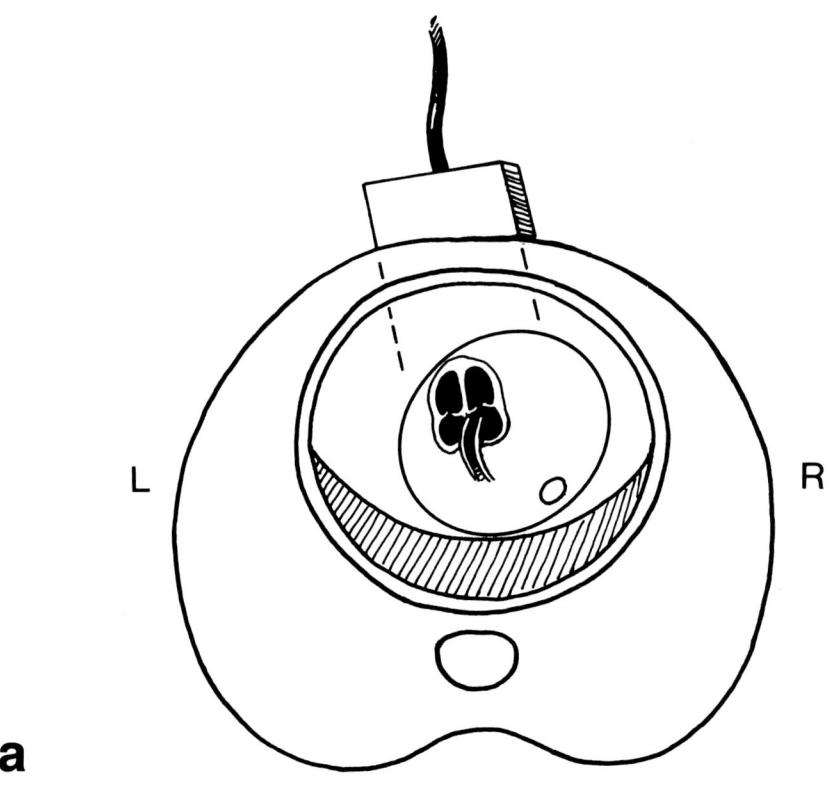

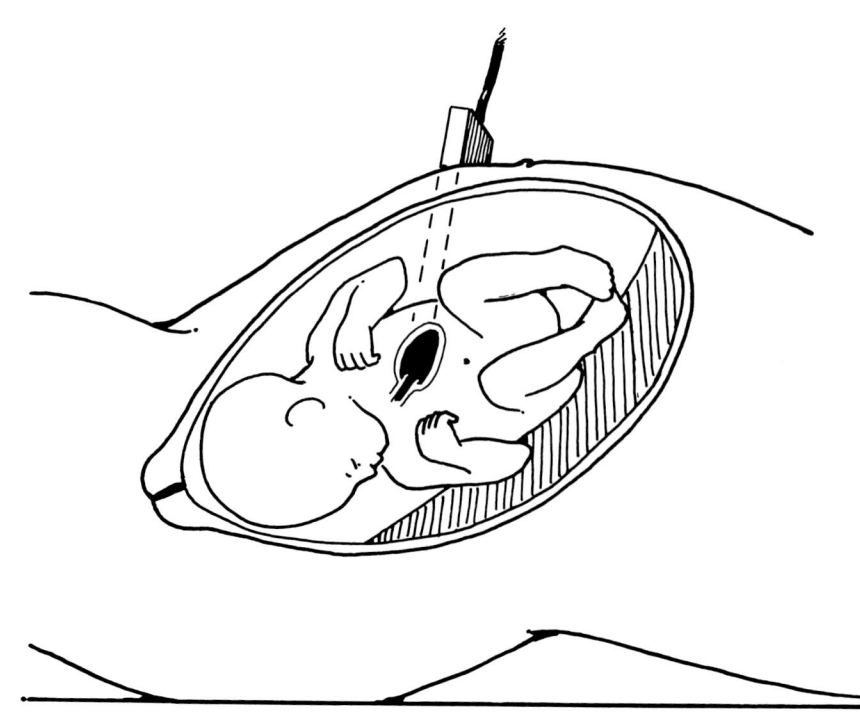

Fig. 3–3a–d. Five-chamber view. The fetus is in a cephalic presentation. The transducer is in the same position as in Figure 3–1 but tilted slightly more toward the fetal head. The ventricular septum forms the right wall of the ascending aorta, and the aorta makes a "fifth chamber" as it passes between the right and left atrium. RV = right ventricle; LV = left ventricle; RA = right atrium; LA = left atrium; AO = aorta; TV = tricuspid valve; MV = mitral valve.

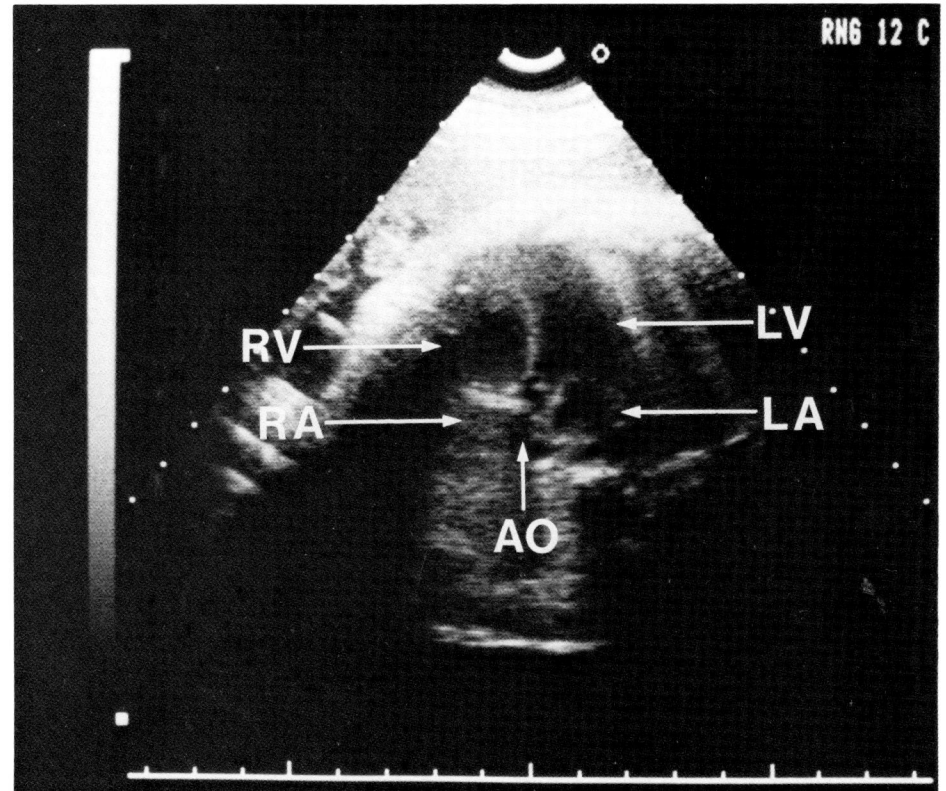

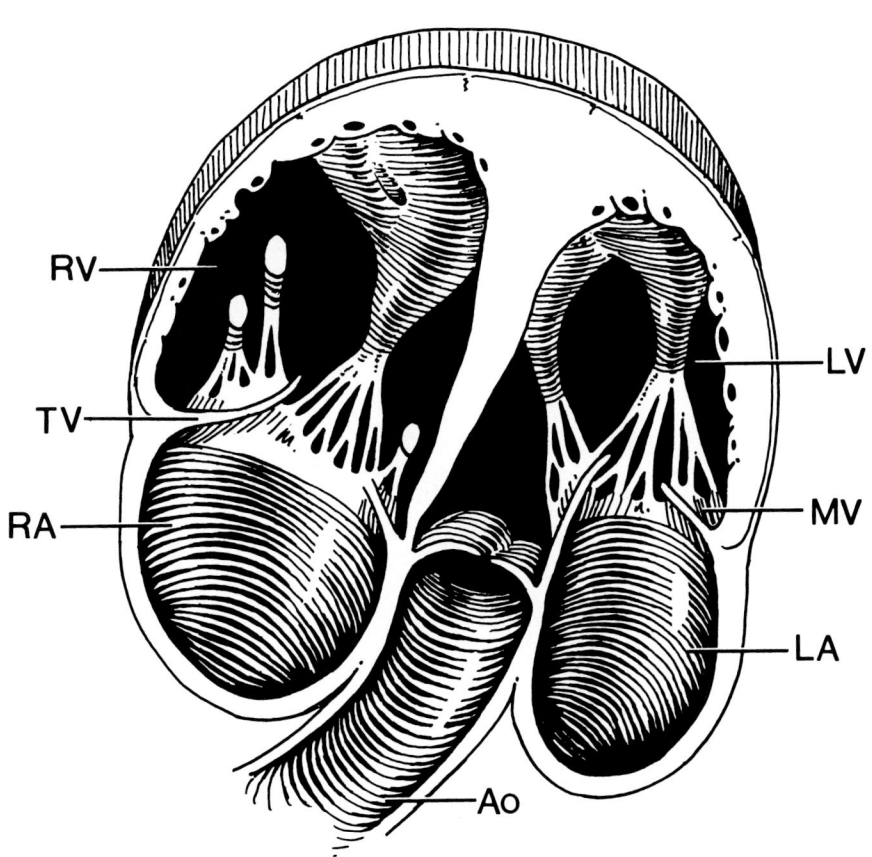

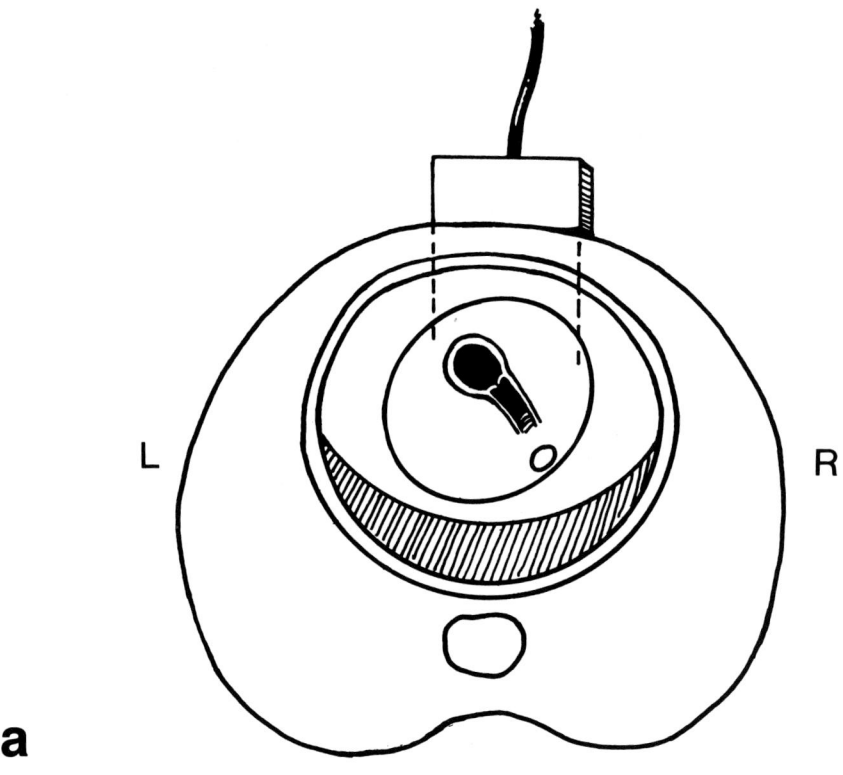

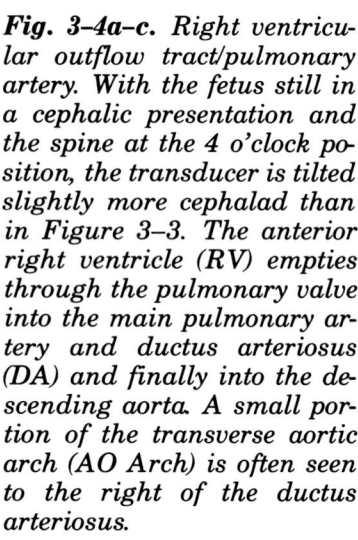

Fig. 3–4a–c. Right ventricular outflow tract/pulmonary artery. With the fetus still in a cephalic presentation and the spine at the 4 o'clock position, the transducer is tilted slightly more cephalad than in Figure 3–3. The anterior right ventricle (RV) empties through the pulmonary valve into the main pulmonary artery and ductus arteriosus (DA) and finally into the descending aorta. A small portion of the transverse aortic arch (AO Arch) is often seen to the right of the ductus arteriosus.

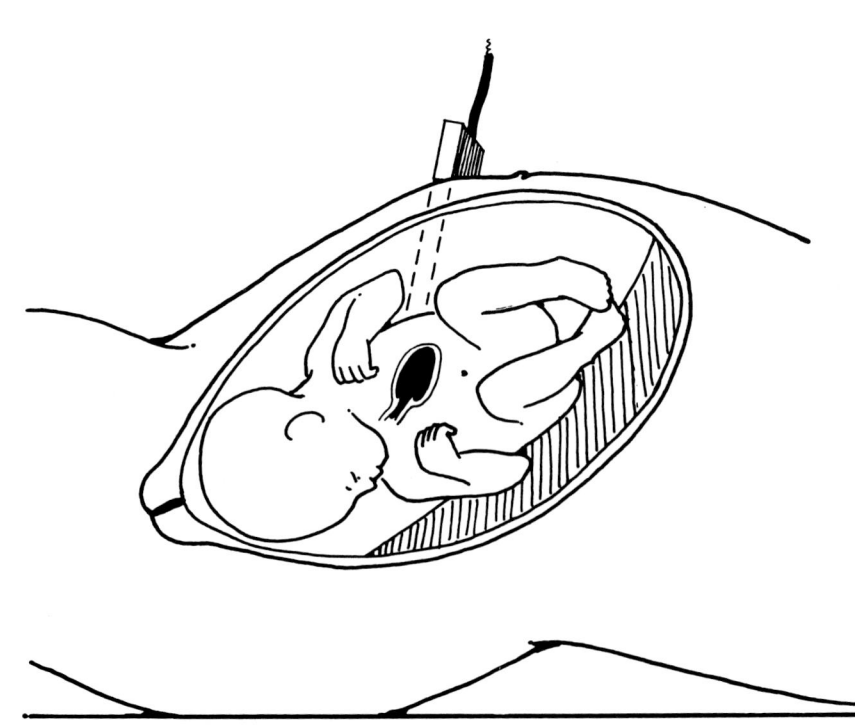

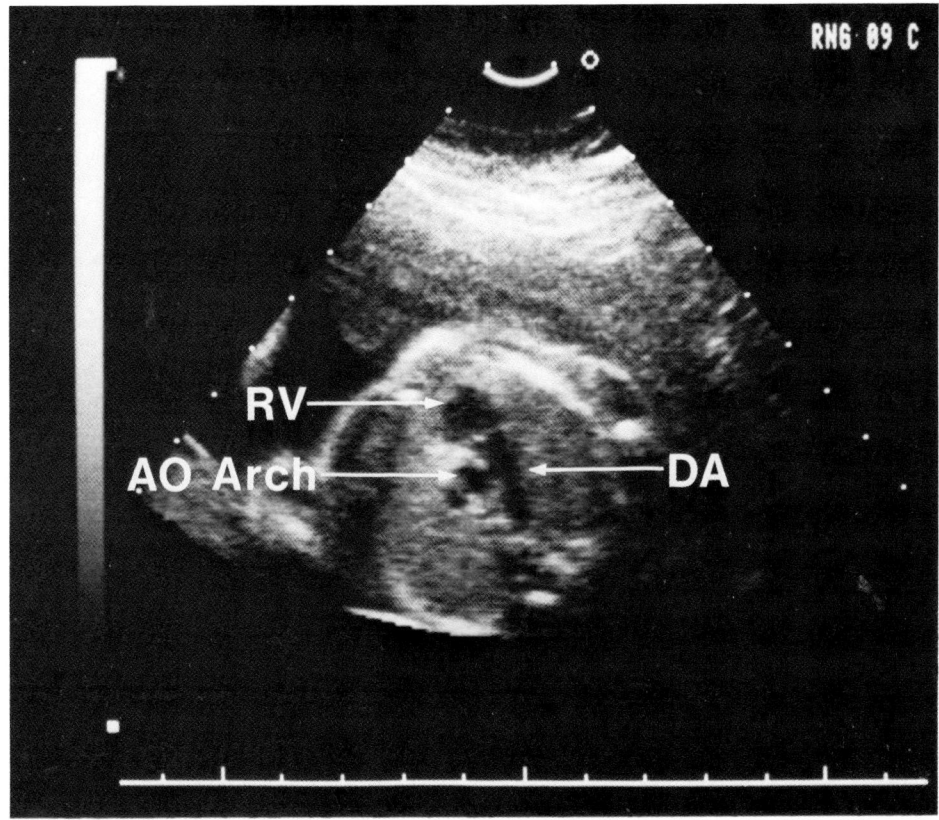

c

LONG AXIS/GREAT VESSEL VIEW

This view is through the long axis of the fetus along the ventral surface. From the apical four-chamber view, rotate the transducer 90 degrees. The apex of the right ventricle is the most anterior structure (Fig. 3–5). The beam transects the right ventricle, the right ventricular outflow tract, and pulmonary artery as it crosses over the ascending aorta. Posterior to the pulmonary artery is the ascending aorta and posterior to the aorta is the superior vena cava. A portion of the tricuspid valve is seen between the right ventricle and right atrium.

Since the inferior vena cava enters the right atrium obliquely to this plane, some right-to-left rotation of the transducer is needed to follow its course posterior to the liver and into the right atrium.

The posterior aspect of this view is through the right posterior chest wall (Fig. 3–6). The right atrium is now the structure closest to the transducer.

The importance of this view rests in the relative positions and sizes of the pulmonary artery and ascending aorta and the sizes and positions of the respective valves.

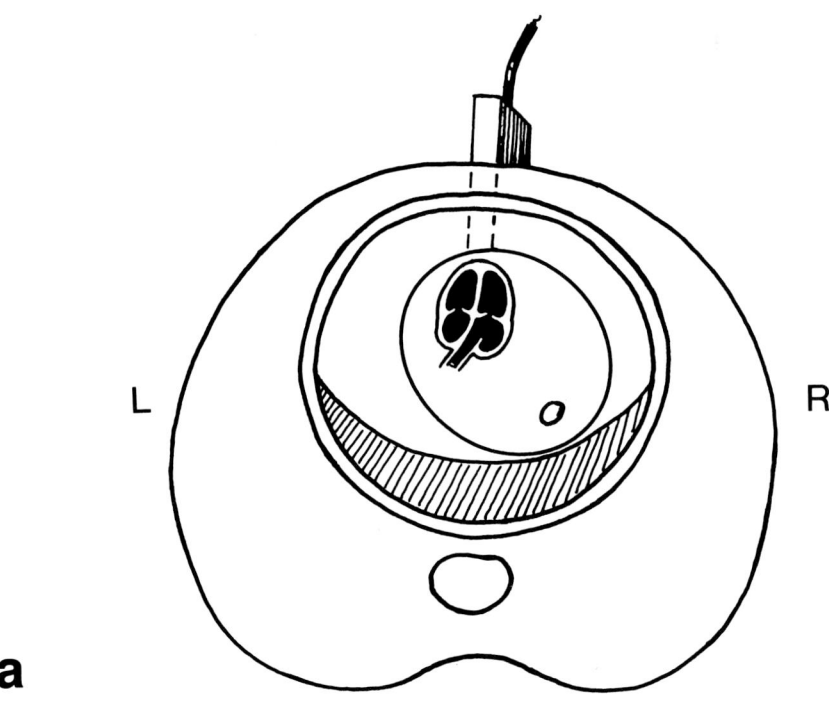

Fig. 3–5 a–d. Long axis/great vessel view. With the fetus in a cephalic presentation and the fetal head at the right of the ultrasound picture, as in Figure 3–1, the transducer has been rotated 90 degrees from the apical four-chamber view. This view transects the right ventricle, the right ventricular outflow tract, and pulmonary artery (PA) as it crosses from right to left anterior to the ascending aorta (AO). Posterior to the aorta, the superior vena cava (SVC) enters the right atrium (RA). The tricuspid valve (TV) is seen inferior to the aortic root. PV = pulmonary valve; RV = right ventricle; AV = aortic valve; IVC = inferior vena cava.

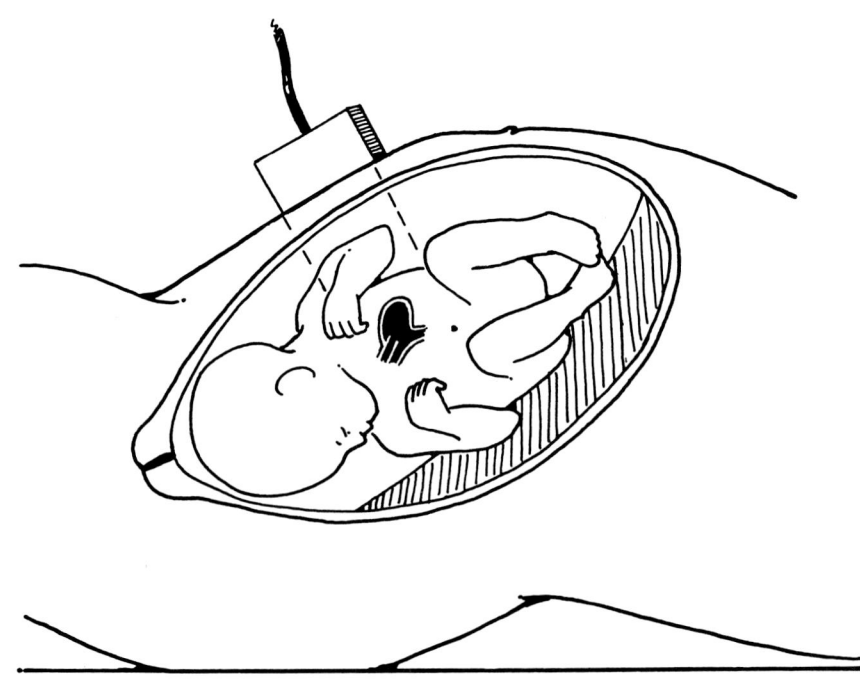

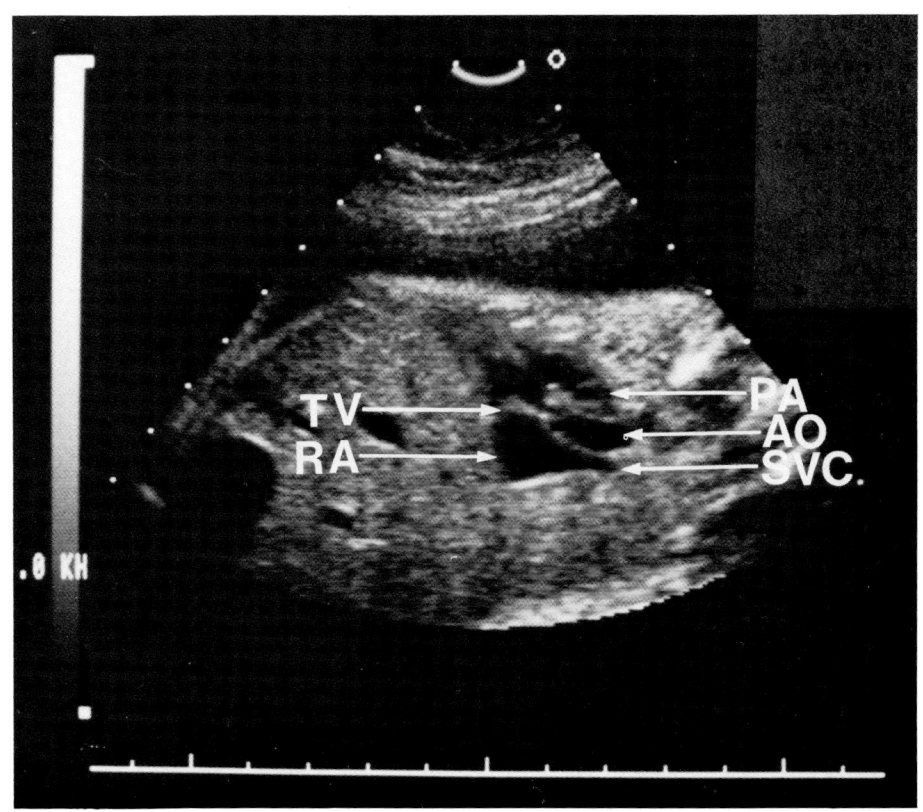

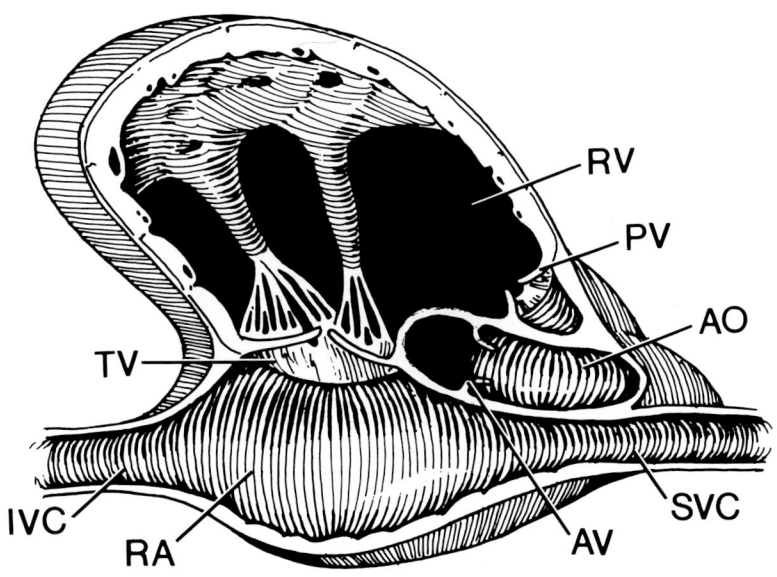

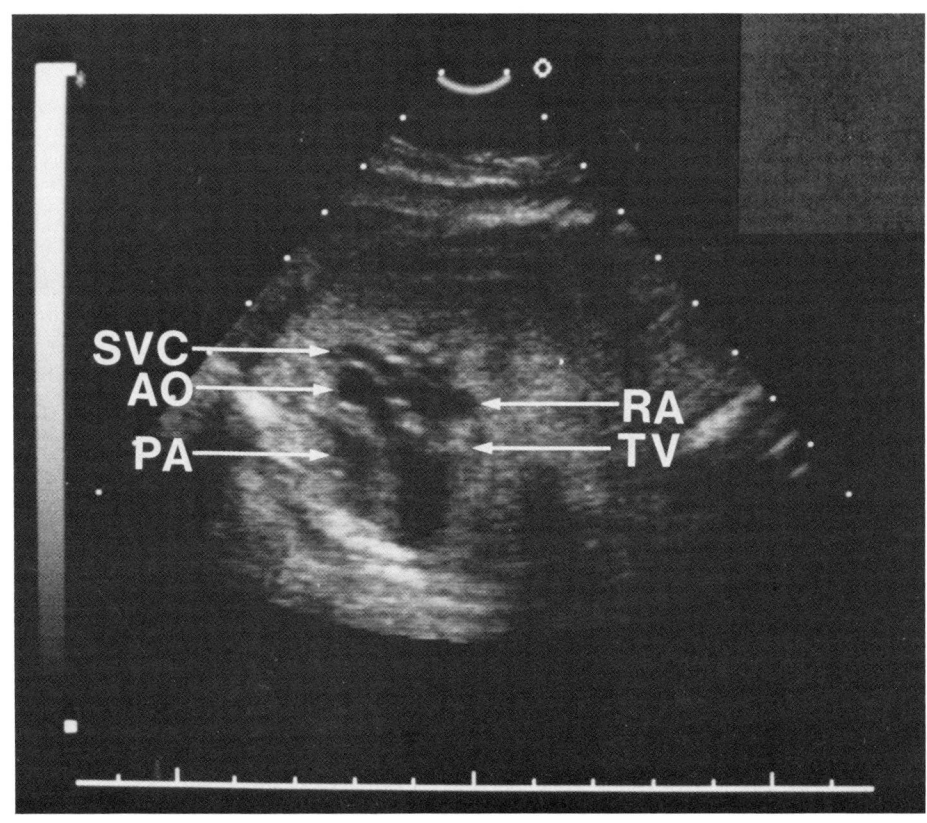

Fig. 3-6a,b. In this view of the great vessels in long axis, the fetus is in a breech presentation with the apex of the fetal heart toward the maternal spine. The fetal head is toward the left of the image. The transducer is positioned across the right posterolateral surface of the fetus. The right atrium (RA), superior vena cava (SVC), and ascending aorta (AO) are seen, along with the pulmonary artery (PA)/right ventricular outflow tract as it crosses the ascending aorta. Part of the tricuspid valve (TV) is seen inferior to the aortic root. AV = aortic valve; IVC = inferior vena cava; PV = pulmonary valve; RV = right ventricle.

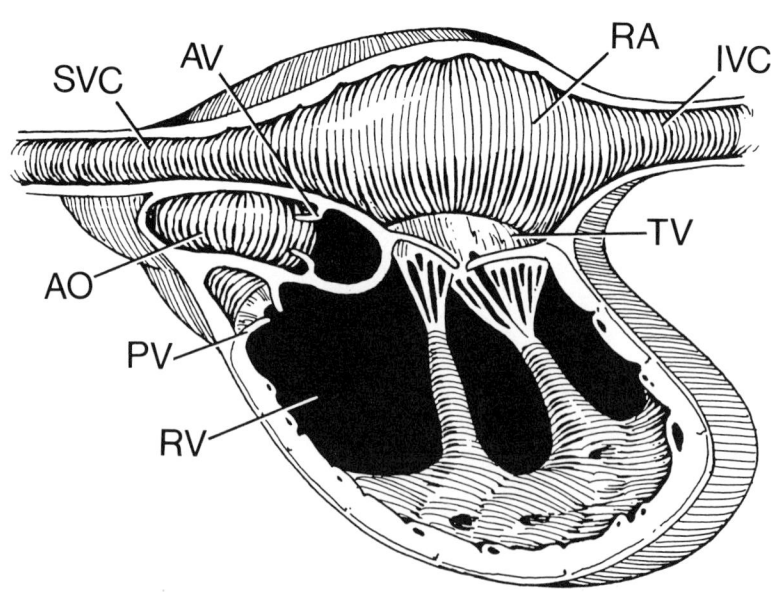

FOUR-CHAMBER/LONG AXIS VIEW

The fetus is in a cephalic presentation, with the fetal spine toward the mother's right. The left ventricle and atrium are closest to the transducer and the fetal spine is between the 1 and 2 o'clock positions (Fig. 3–7). As the title infers, this cross section is taken through the long axis of the heart, transecting the left lateral chest wall. All four chambers and ventricular and atrial septae are perpendicular to the ultrasound beam. Fractional shortening measurements of the ventricles in systole and diastole can be obtained from this view. Because of problems with lateral resolution, this view may be less accurate for diagnosis of septal defects than the near-parallel apical four-chamber view. This view is excellent for measurements of cardiac wall thickness, septal thickness, and chamber sizes. The pulmonary veins can be seen entering the left atrium in this view. The flap of the foramen ovale is present in the left atrium.

LEFT VENTRICULAR OUTFLOW TRACT/LONG AXIS

From the four-chamber/long axis view, the transducer is angled slightly cephalad, revealing the anterior portion of the left ventricle, the aortic root, the aortic valve, and the ascending aorta (Fig. 3–8). A small portion of the right ventricle and the right atrium is also seen. The ventricular septum is contiguous with the medial wall of the aorta. The ascending aorta arises from the midportion of the heart and courses anteriorly and to the right within the fetal thorax.

Because the ultrasound beam encounters the ventricular septum at a right angle rather than close to parallel, lateral resolution makes it difficult to rule out a small but significant defect. An overriding aorta or narrowing of any portion of the ascending aorta can be determined from this view.

RIGHT VENTRICULAR OUTFLOW TRACT/LONG AXIS

By sliding the transducer slightly toward the fetal head, the right ventricular outflow tract can be seen, including the superior portion of the right ventricle, the pulmonary valve, the main pulmonary artery, and the ductus arteriosus as it enters the descending aorta anterior to the spine (Fig. 3–9). The right ventricular outflow tract crosses from the right anterior portion of the thorax to the left posterior region. A lateral view of the transverse aortic arch is seen to the right of the main pulmonary artery and proximal portion of the ductus.

Both of these long axis views of the aorta and pulmonary artery, lying in close proximity to one another, allow the examiner to easily see their relationships by "rocking" the tranducer back and forth. Transposition of the great vessels can sometimes be detected using this maneuver. Double outlet of the right ventricle, and aortic and pulmonic stenosis and atresia can also be detected utilizing these views (Tables 3–3 and 3–4).

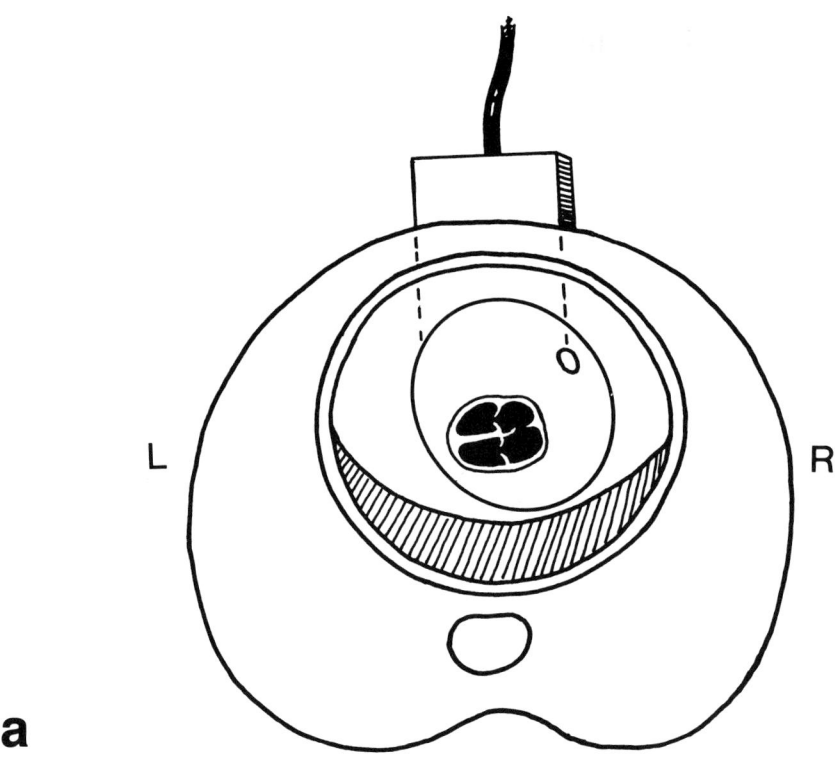

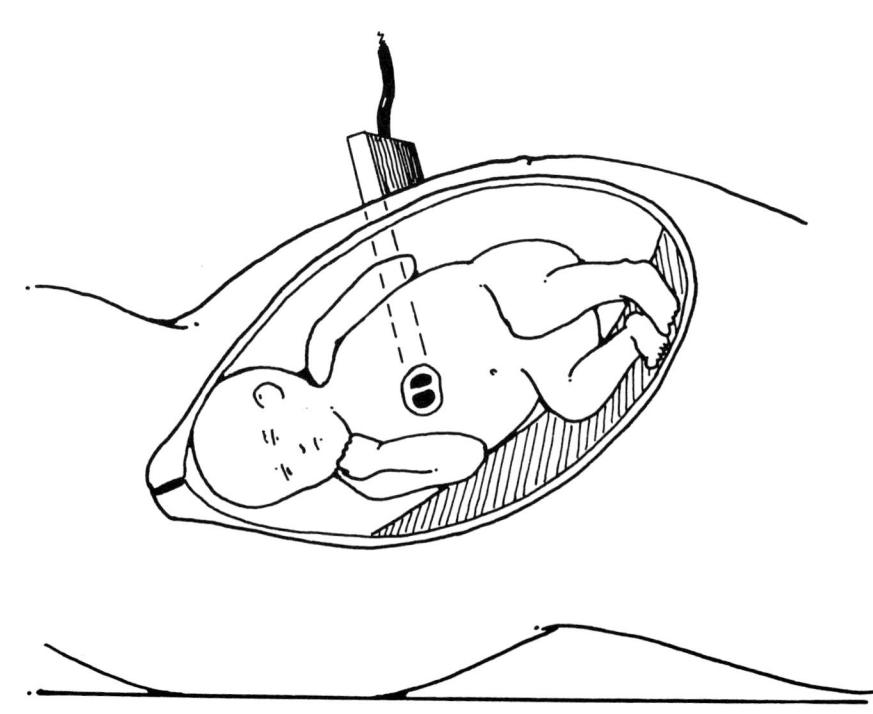

Fig. 3-7a-d. Four-chamber/long axis view. With the fetus in a cephalic presentation and the spine at the 2 o'clock position, all four chambers of the fetal heart are seen in long axis with the ventricular septum perpendicular to the ultrasound beam. Cardiac wall thickness, septal thickness, and papillary muscles as well as chamber diameters during systole and diastole, both atrioventricular valves, foramen ovale (FO) and flap, and pulmonary veins (PVn) are seen in this view. M-mode tracings of this view are utilized for chamber diameter, septal, and wall measurements. RV = right ventricle; LV = left ventricle; RA = right atrium; LA = left atrium; MV = mitral valve; TV = tricuspid valve; SV = superior vena cava.

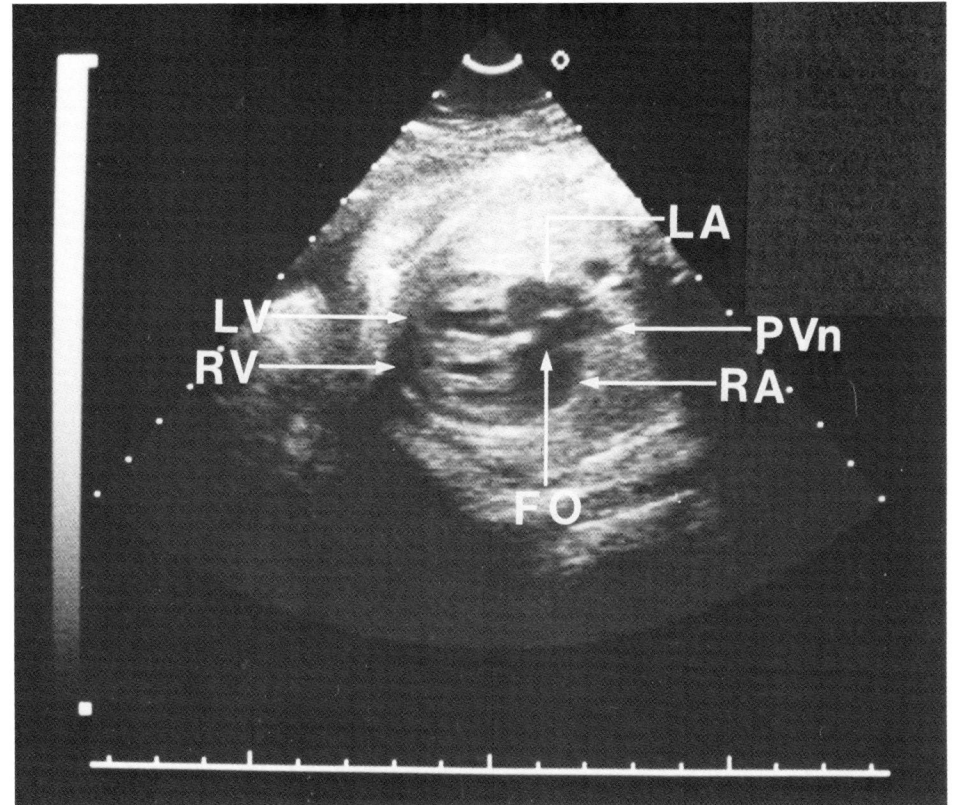

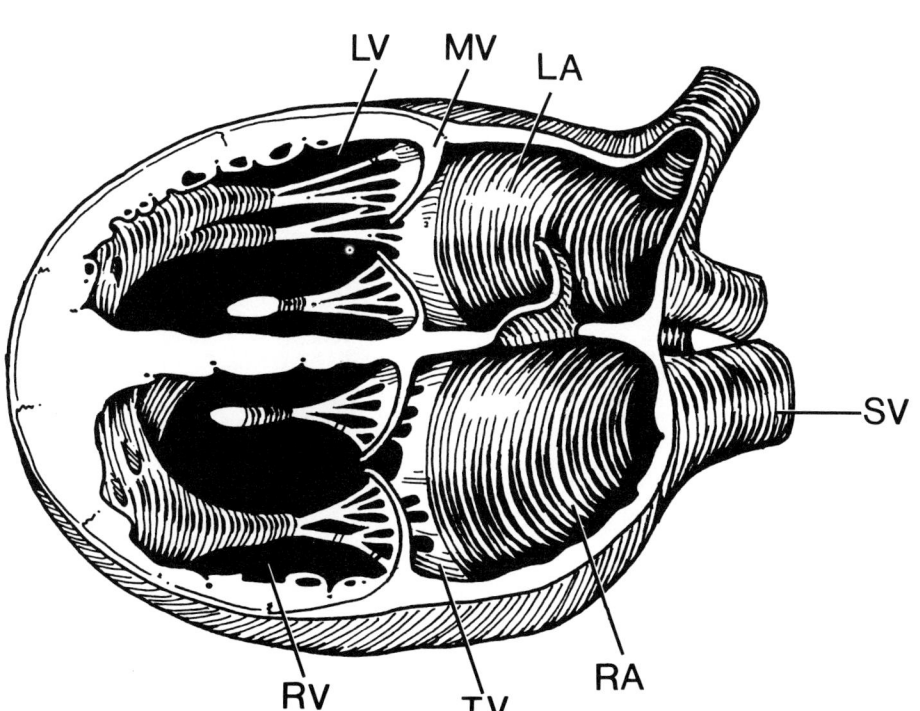

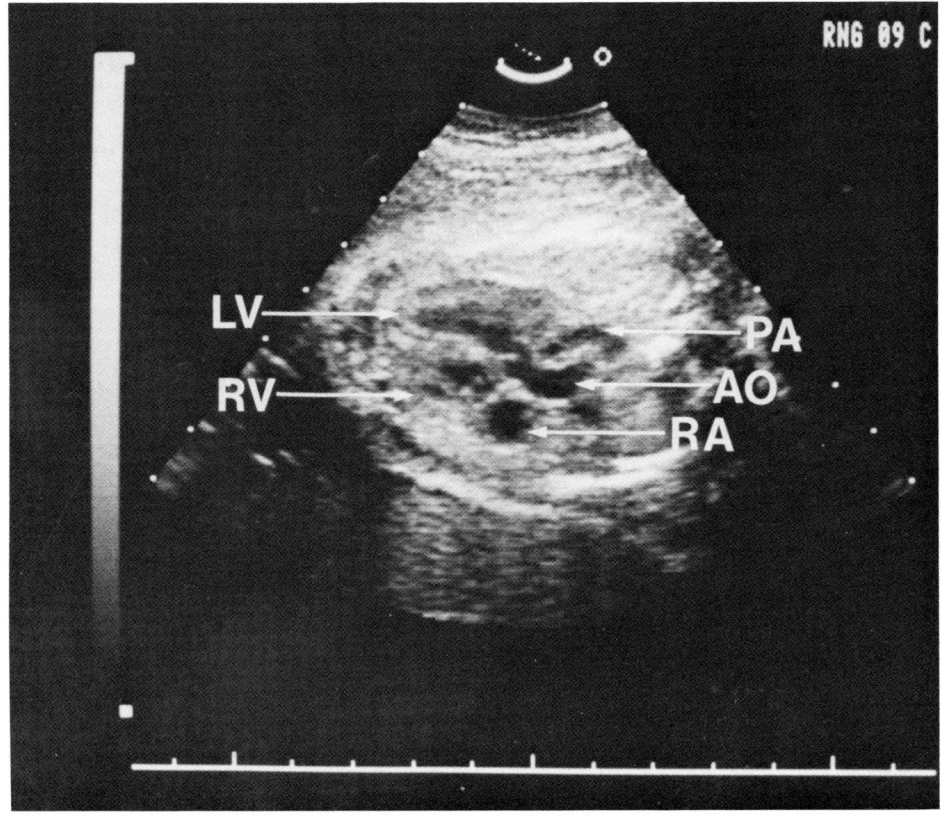

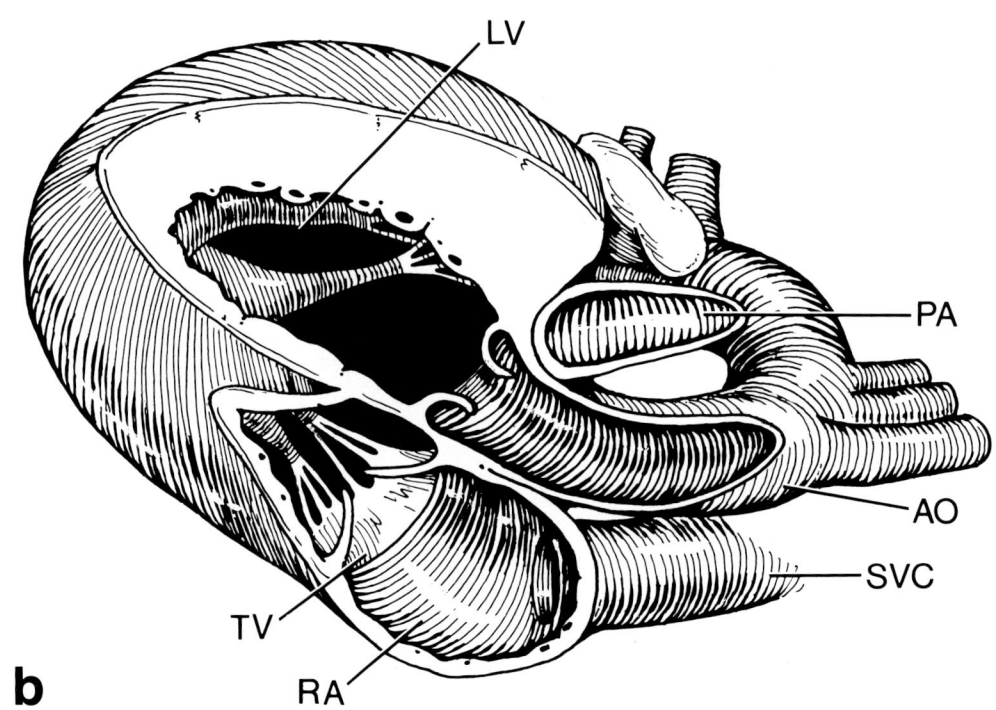

Fig. 3-8a,b. Left ventricular outflow tract/long axis. From Figure 3-7, the transducer is tilted toward the fetal head. The ascending aorta (AO) can be seen arising from the left ventricle (LV). The ventricular septum forms the right wall of the aorta. The aorta originates centrally within the heart and exits from left to right and superiorly and then bends back to the left to form the transverse arch, which cannot be seen from this view. RV = right ventricle; PA = pulmonary artery; RA = right atrium; TV = tricuspid valve; SVC = superior vena cava.

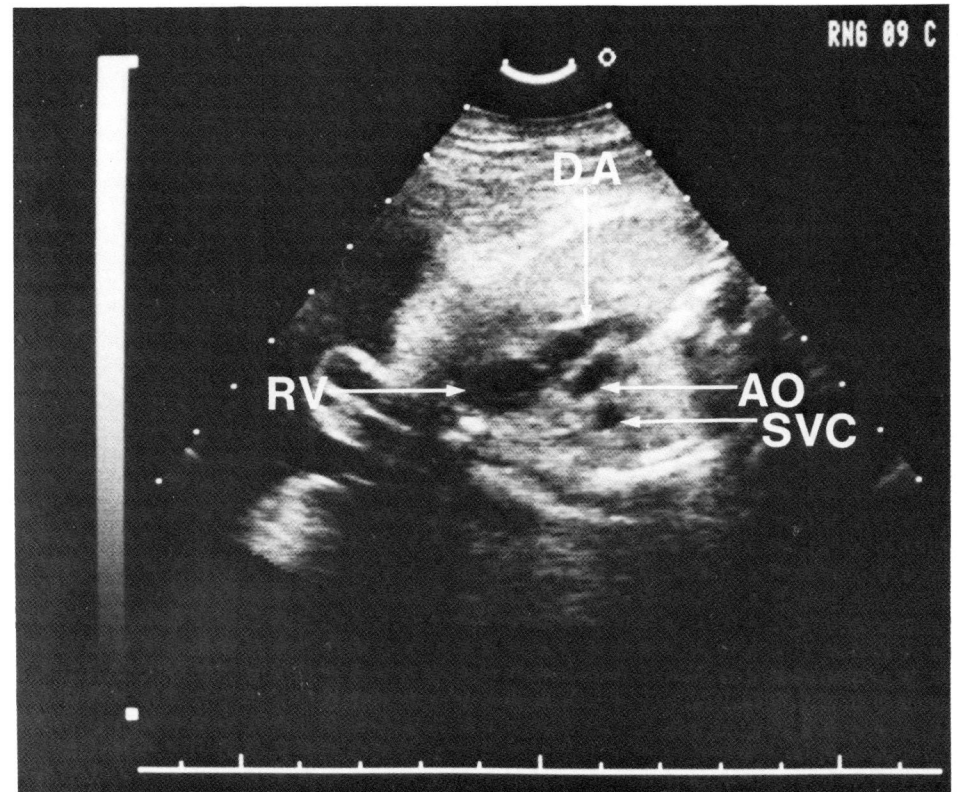

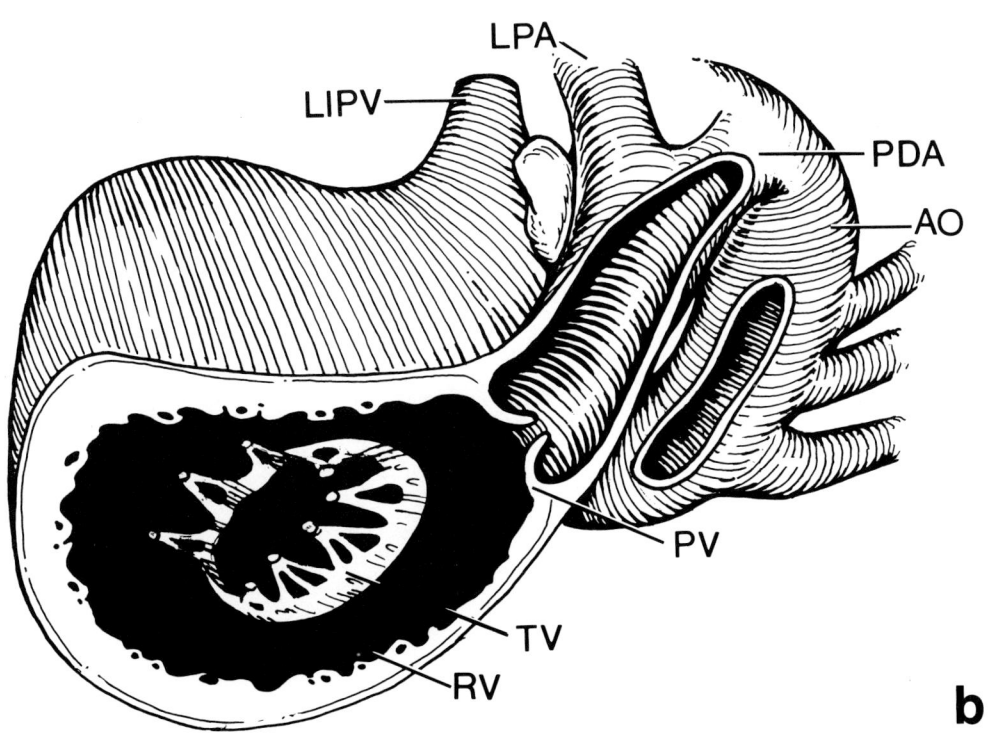

Fig. 3-9a,b. Right ventricular outflow tract /long axis. The transducer is moved slightly more toward the fetal head from the transducer position in Figure 3-8. This view exhibits the superior portion of the right ventricle (RV) as it exits through the pulmonary valve into the main pulmonary artery and ductus arteriosus (DA). A small portion of the transverse aortic arch (AO) lies to the right of the main pulmonary artery and ductus arteriosus. A cross section of the superior vena cava (SVC) is seen to the right and posterior to the transverse arch. PDA = patent ductus arteriosus; LPA = left pulmonary artery; LIPV = left inferior pulmonary vein; TV = tricuspid valve; PV = pulmonary valve.

TABLE 3-3. Basic Anatomy: Great Vessels

Pulmonary artery is about 20% larger than ascending aorta

Pulmonary artery/ductal arch	Ascending aorta/aortic arch
Begins anteriorly	Begins centrally
Crosses right to left	Crosses left to right
Makes a wider curve	Makes a tighter curve
Position is lower in chest	Position is higher in chest
	Vessels exit to head

TABLE 3-4. Fetal Cardiac Anatomy: Great Vessels

Long axis/great vessel	Short axis/great vessel
Structures seen	
Pulmonary valve	Pulmonary valve
Main pulmonary artery	Main pulmonary artery
Aortic valve/ascending aorta	Right pulmonary artery
Superior/inferior vena cava	Aorta (cross section)
Right atrium	
Tricuspid valve	

Measurements
Compare great vessel sizes

Anomalies ruled out
Valve atresia/stenosis/insufficiency
Transposition of the great vessels
Tetralogy of Fallot
Truncus arteriosus

TABLE 3-5. Fetal Cardiac Anatomy: Great Vessel Arches

Pulmonary artery/ductal arch	Ascending aorta/aortic arch
Structures seen	
Pulmonary valve	Aortic valve (rarely)
Main pulmonary artery	Ascending aorta
Ductus insertion	Transverse arch
Cross section of aorta	Vessels exit to head
Descending aorta	Descending aorta

Anomalies ruled out
Valve atresia/stenosis/insufficiency
Premature closure of the ductus
Coarctation of the aorta

TRANSVENTRICULAR VIEW

In this view the beam transects the long axis of the fetus in a transverse cross section of the heart (Fig. 3–10). With the transducer in position for the long axis, four-chamber view, rotate transducer 90 degrees, and position the transducer so that the beam transects the right or left anterolateral chest wall passing to the opposite anterolateral chest wall of the fetus. This procedure will produce a cross section of the heart from the apex to the base as the transducer is moved from the ventral to the dorsal side of the fetus. Placing the transducer nearer the ventral aspect of the fetus will produce an image of the ventricles in short axis cross section. This view will allow the examiner to evaluate ventricular walls, the ventricular septum, papillary muscle positions, and ventricular chamber shapes and sizes.

As the transducer is moved toward the dorsal side of the fetus, the ventricular septum becomes thinner, and the tricuspid and mitral valve leaflets begin to appear during their excursions throughout the cardiac cycle. M-mode tracings can be made just below valve leaflet attachments for the purpose of measuring ventricular diameters, cardiac wall thickness, and septal thickness during systole and diastole.

SHORT AXIS/GREAT VESSEL VIEW

This view is important because it shows the relationship of the great vessels.

When the fetus is in a sternum anterior position, this view is obtained by placing the transducer so that the beam makes a transverse cross section of the upper portion of the anterior chest wall of the fetus with a caudal tilt of the transducer (Figs. 3–11 and 3–12). This position is slightly inferior to a suprasternal approach with a small counterclockwise rotation. The beam should transect the right ventricular outflow tract as it exits the right ventricle, the pulmonary valve, the main pulmonary artery, the ductus arteriosus, and the right pulmonary artery. The ductus arteriosus joins the descending aorta anterior to the spine. The main pulmonary artery and right pulmonary artery wrap around the ascending aorta creating an image that looks like a "doughnut." The caudal portion of this image is made up of the right ventricle, tricuspid valve, and right atrium.

The importance of this view lies in the relative positions and origins of the great vessels as well as their diameters (Table 3–4).

If the examiner is approaching the fetus through the right lateral chest wall, the transducer should be positioned nearer the fetal diaphragm and tilted cephalad.

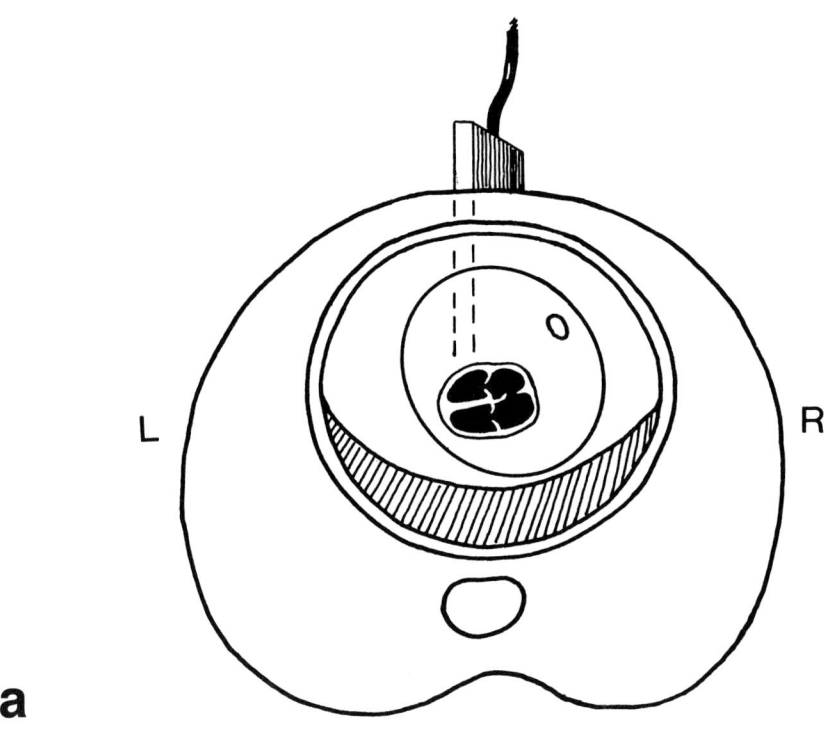

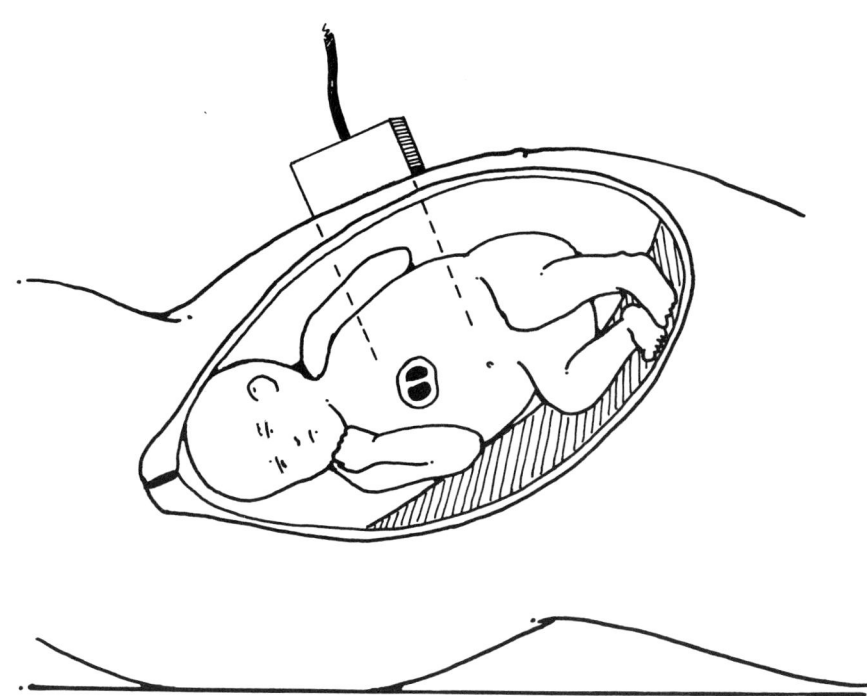

Fig. 3-10a-d. Transventricular view. From the four-chamber/long axis view as seen in Figure 3-7, the transducer is rotated 90 degrees so that the ventricles and atria can be seen in short axis cross section. Chamber shapes, cardiac walls, and the septum and papillary muscles (PM) can be seen. RV = right ventricle; LV = left ventricle.

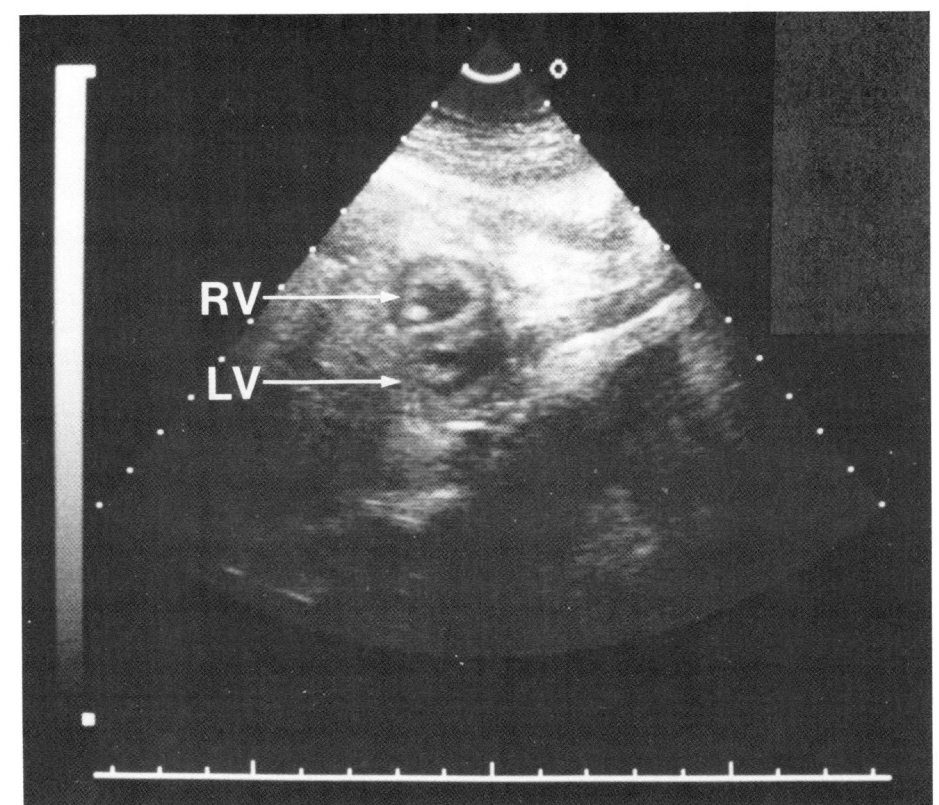

c

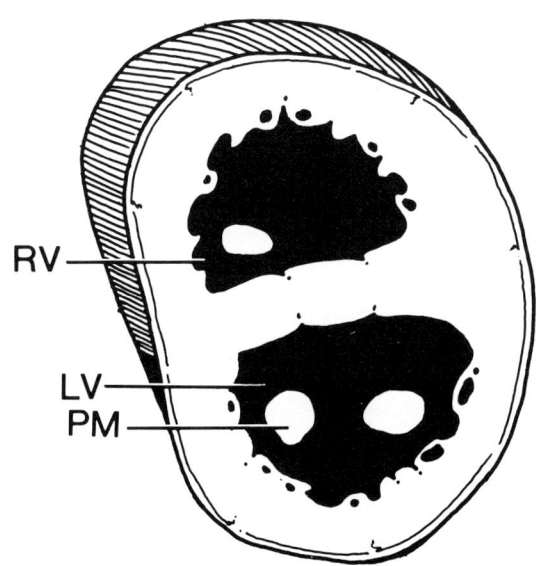

d

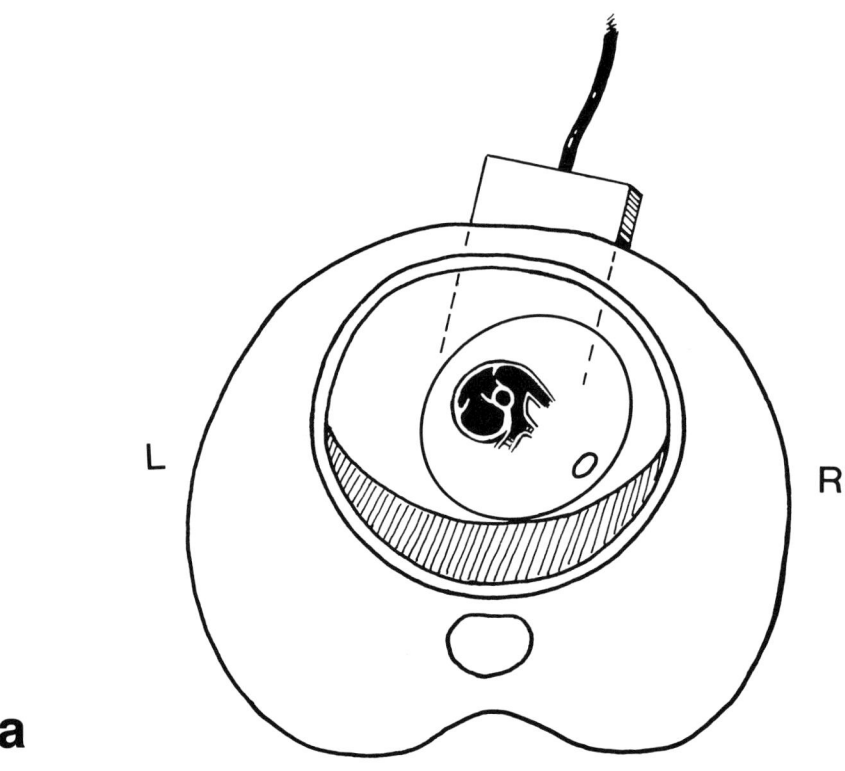

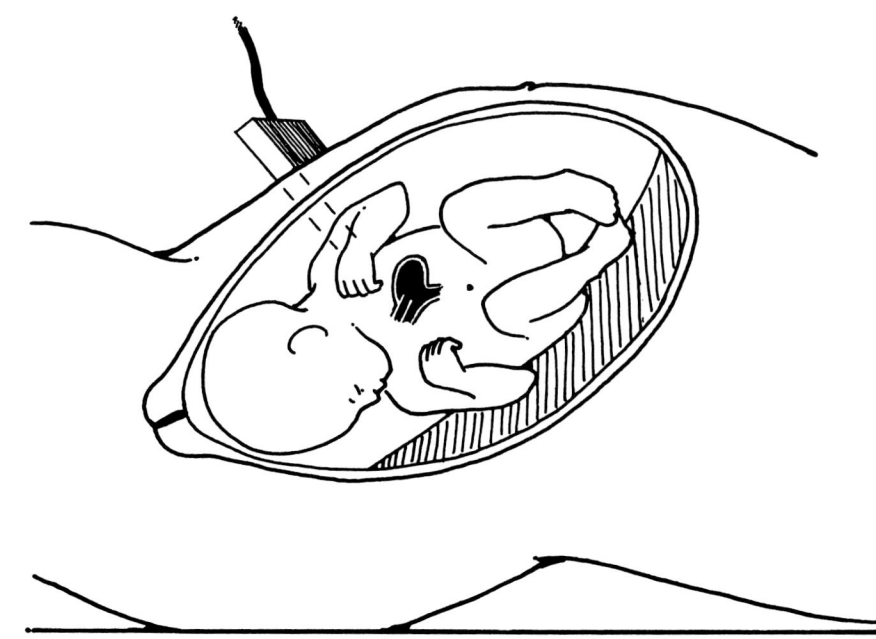

Fig. 3-11a-d. Short axis/great vessel view. This fetus is in a cephalic presentation with the spine at the 2 o'clock position. Whereas in Figure 3-12 the view is obtained by tilting the transducer cephalad from the inferior fetal thorax, in this view the transducer is tilted caudally from just below the fetal neck. In the diagram, the fetal spine is shown in the 4 o'clock position. PV = pulmonary valve; DA = ductus arteriosus; RPA = right pulmonary artery; AO = aorta; TV = tricuspid valve; Desc AO = descending aorta; LPA = left pulmonary artery; RV = right ventricle.

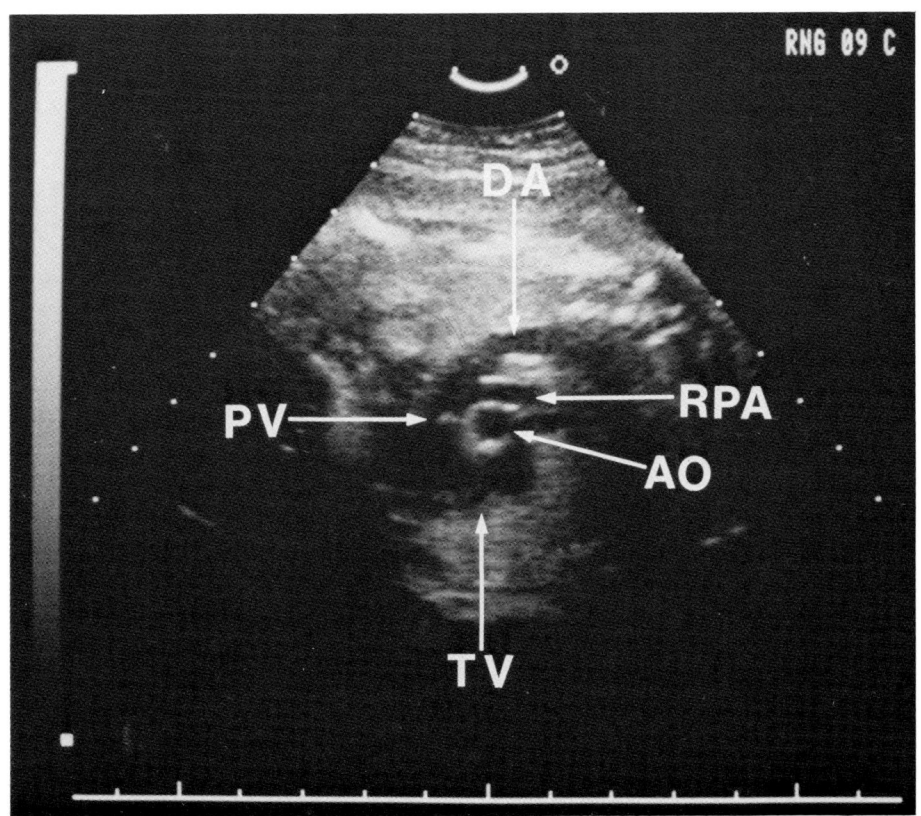

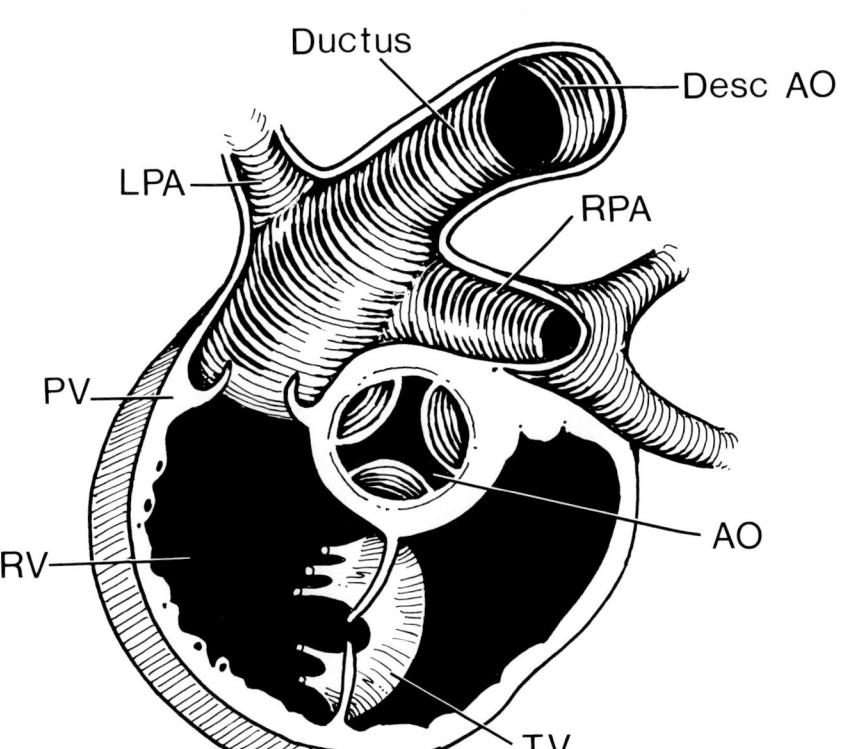

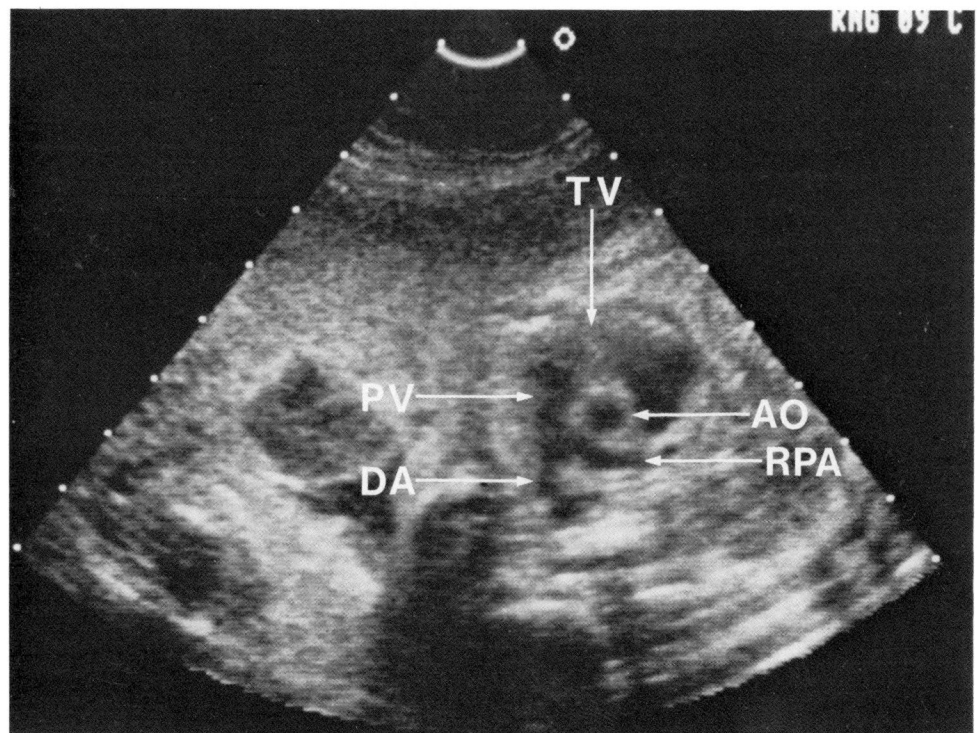

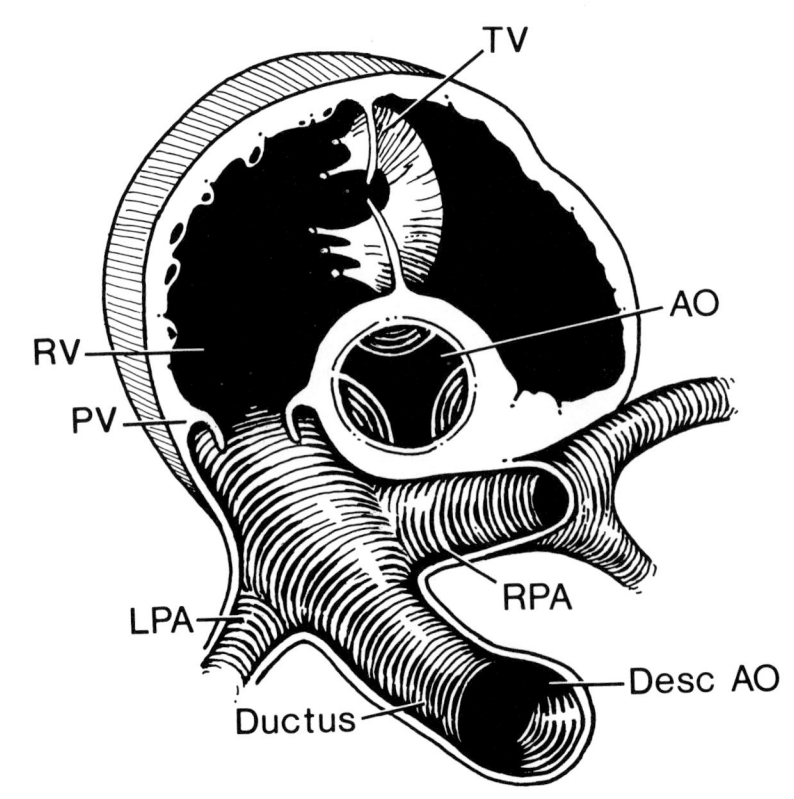

Fig. 3-12a,b. Short axis/great vessel view. The fetus is in a breech presentation with the spine at the 6 o'clock position. This view has a "doughnut" appearance created by the right atrium and right ventricle (RV), which form one side, and the main pulmonary artery and right pulmonary artery (RPA), which wrap around the ascending aorta (AO) to form the opposite side of the outer circle. The main pulmonary artery becomes the ductus arteriosus (DA) immediately after the bifurcation with the right pulmonary artery and empties into the descending aorta (Desc AO) anterior to the spine. PV = pulmonary valve; TV = tricuspid valve; LPA = left pulmonary artery.

AORTIC ARCH

The ascending aorta, arising from the left ventricle, crosses initially from left to right, passing behind the pulmonary artery. It then bends from right to left and courses slightly anteriorly as it becomes the transverse arch. At this point, the transverse arch lies adjacent and slightly superior to the ductus arteriosus. It then curves posteriorly and inferiorly and becomes the descending portion of the aorta. Because of this somewhat tortuous course, the entire aorta from root to descending portion cannot be seen in one single view.

The easiest technique for examining the aortic arch and descending aorta is to place the transducer along the long axis of the fetus to the left of the fetal spine (Fig. 3–13). The beam should transect the left posterior chest wall and exit the right lateral chest wall. A small portion of the left and right atria may be seen anterior and posterior to the ascending portion of the aorta. The left subclavian artery, left common carotid artery, and the brachiocephalic trunk, should be visible arising from the transverse arch (Figs. 3–13 and 3–14).

If the fetal spine is posterior (Fig. 3–14), the transducer is placed so that the beam will enter the right lateral chest wall looking toward the left posterior chest wall.

This view is important in the diagnosis of transposition of the great vessels and coarctation of the aorta (Table 3–5).

DUCTAL ARCH

Whereas the aortic arch has been described as a "candy cane" in shape, the ductal arch has been described as a "hockey stick," since it originates anterior to the aorta and has a much broader curve. The ductus arteriosus enters the descending aorta superior to the point at which the transverse arch becomes the descending aorta (Fig. 3–15).

The ductal arch is more easily appreciated from the ventral surface of the fetus in a longitudinal cross section, since it is usually obscured by the fetal spine from the dorsal surface, especially late in gestation. The transducer is placed so that the beam enters the fetal thorax to the right of the sternum and transects the thorax slightly toward the left as it passes through the chest. The descending aorta is seen anterior to the spine; the ductus arteriosus enters it in a smooth curve. There should be no evidence of cerebral vessels along the superior aspect of this arch. The trachea and esophagus lie in close proximity and are often fluid filled but can be ruled out as cerebral vessels, since they do not pulsate as the arteries do (Fig. 3–16).

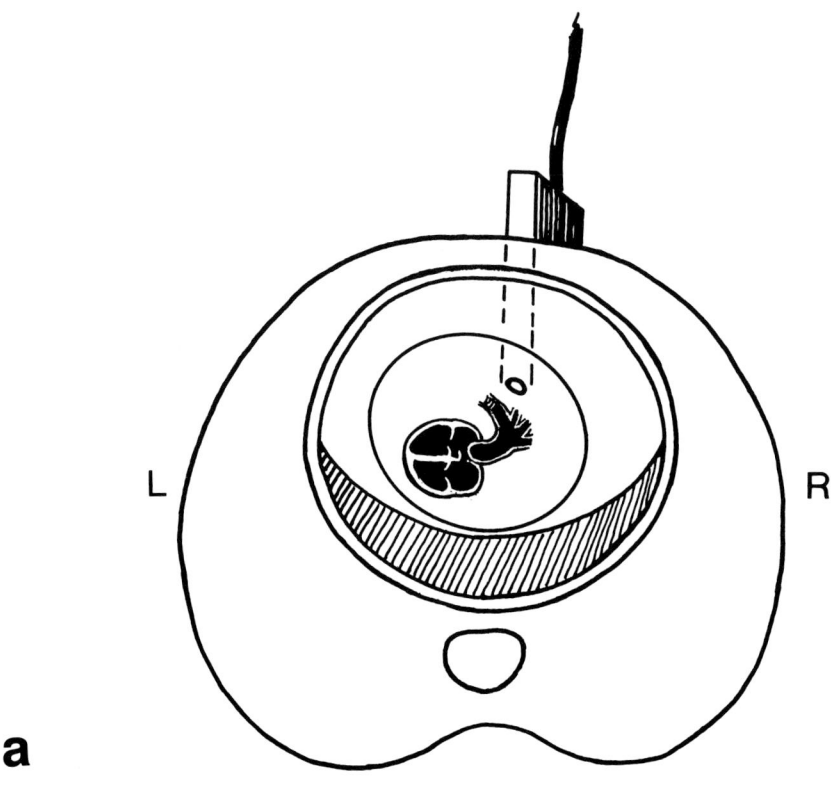

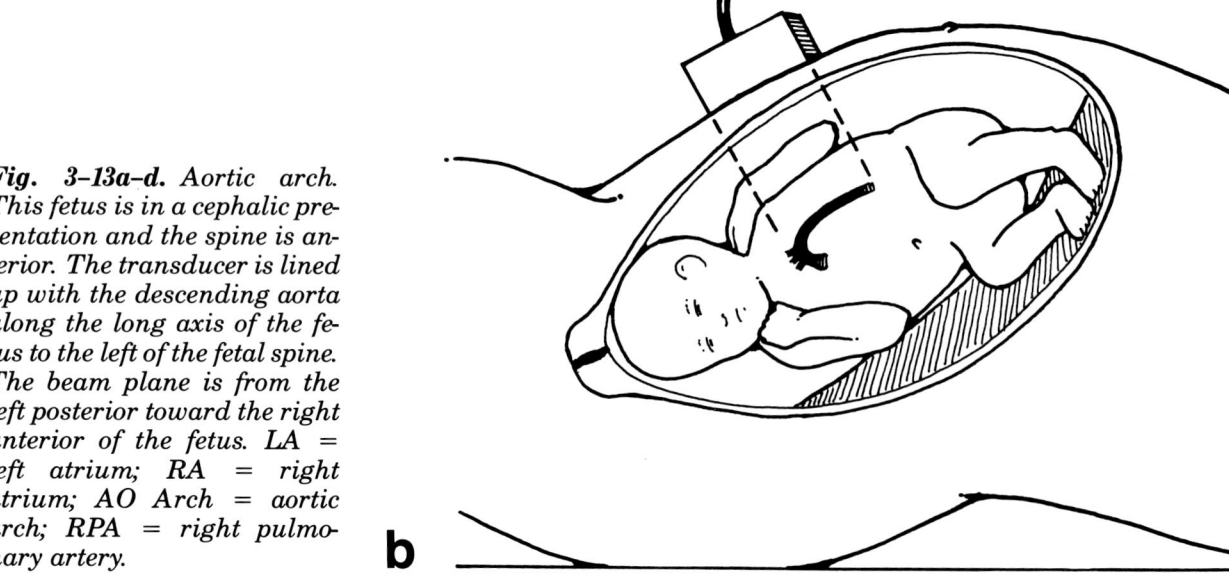

Fig. 3-13a-d. Aortic arch. This fetus is in a cephalic presentation and the spine is anterior. The transducer is lined up with the descending aorta along the long axis of the fetus to the left of the fetal spine. The beam plane is from the left posterior toward the right anterior of the fetus. LA = left atrium; RA = right atrium; AO Arch = aortic arch; RPA = right pulmonary artery.

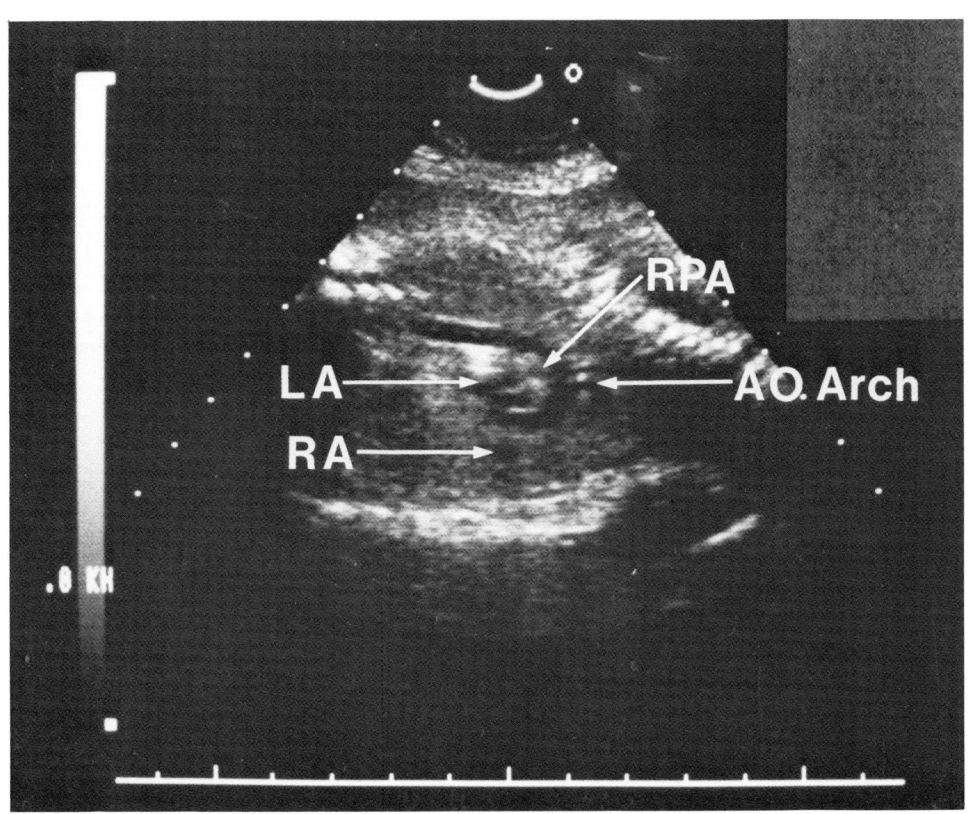

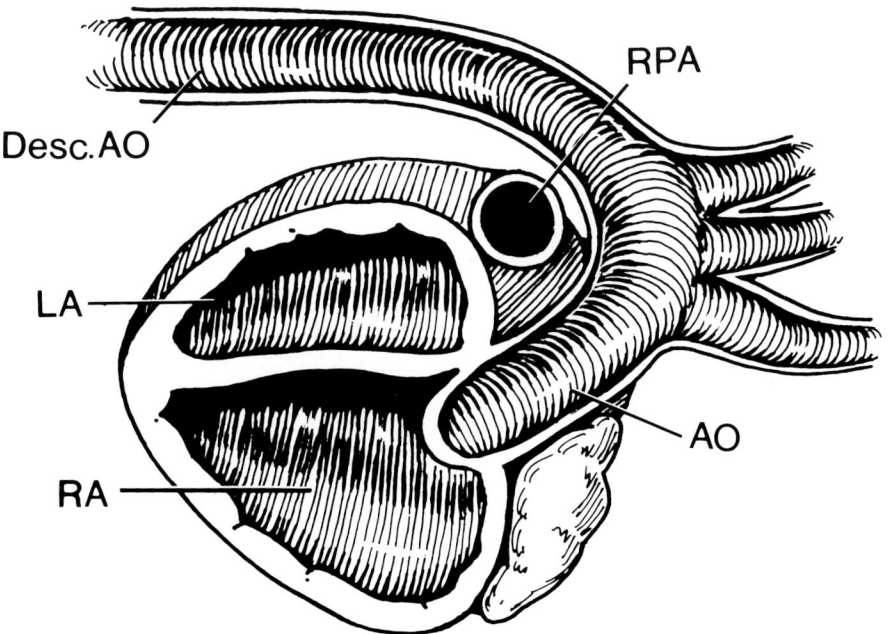

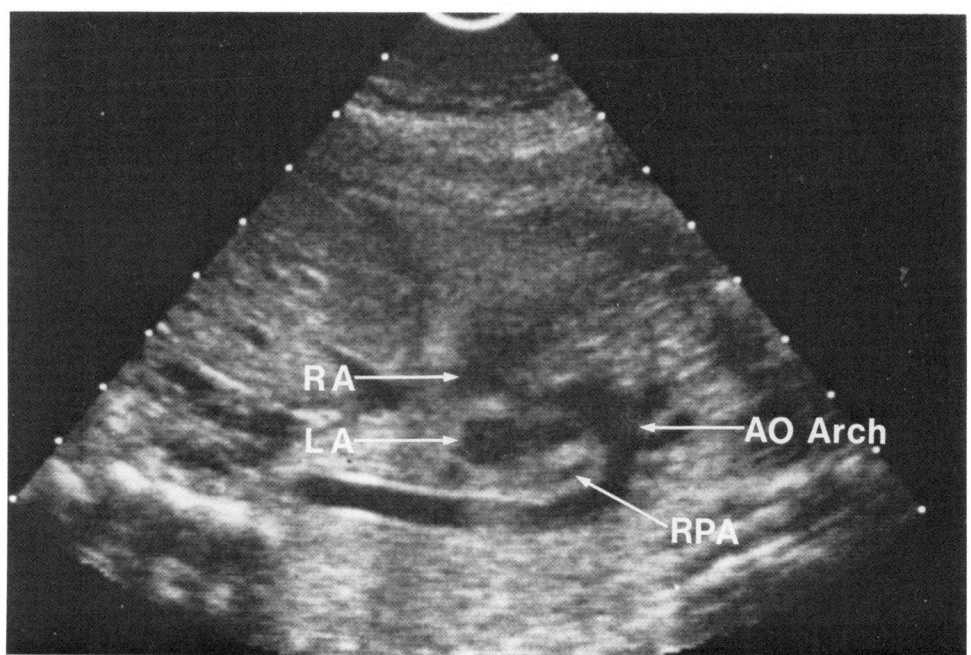

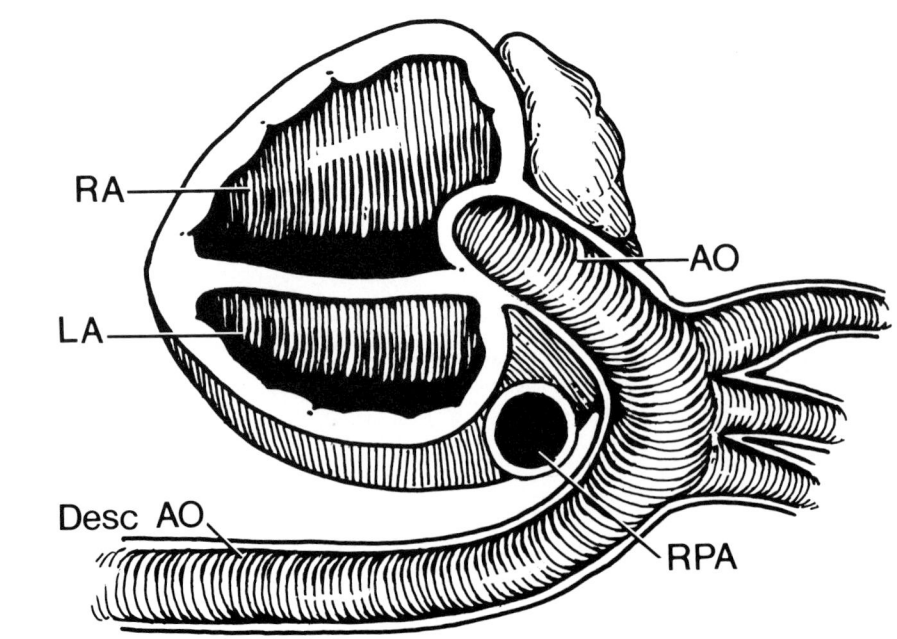

Fig. 3-14a,b. Aortic arch. The fetus is in a cephalic presentation with the spine posterior. A small portion of the ascending aorta is seen as it becomes the transverse arch after it arises from between the left (LA) and right (RA) atria. The acute curve of the transverse arch (AO Arch) gives the structure a "candy cane" appearance, with the cerebral vessels arising from the superior aspect of the arch. The right pulmonary artery (RPA) is seen anterior to the region where the transverse arch curves inferiorly to become the descending aorta (Desc AO).

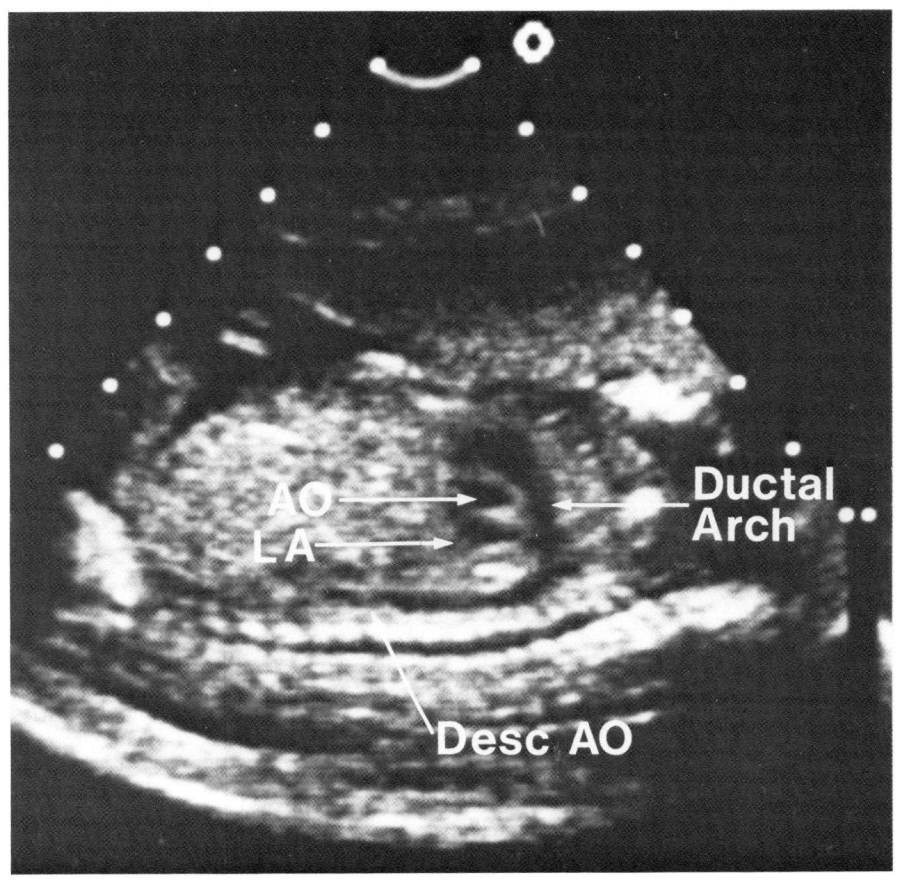

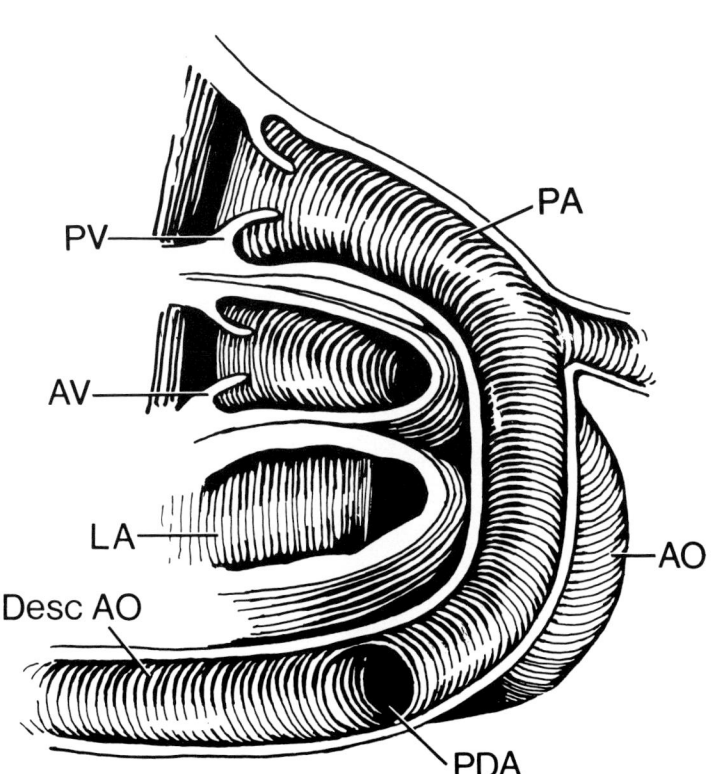

Fig. 3-15a,b. Ductal arch. This structure has been described as having a "hockey stick" appearance because of its broad curve. Unlike the aortic arch, which can be seen from either ventral or dorsal surface of the fetus, the ductal arch is difficult to see from the dorsal surface since its position is more directly anterior to the spine than is the aortic arch. The ductal arch is seen in the long axis of the fetus and is comprised of the right ventricle and main pulmonary artery (PA) coursing directly posteriorly, forming the ductus arteriosus (PDA), which finally curves to enter the descending aorta (Desc AO). No vessels should be seen arising from the superior aspect of this arch. The left pulmonary artery may be seen exiting from the main pulmonary artery. AO = aorta; LA = left atrium; PV = pulmonary valve; AV = aortic valve.

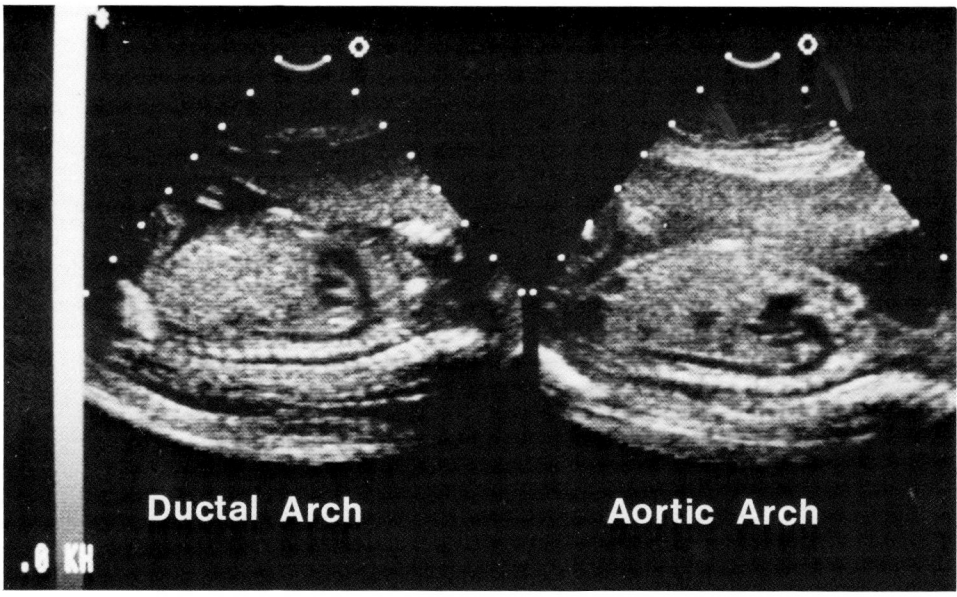

Fig. 3-16. This image shows the fetus in a cephalic presentation with the spine posterior. The ductal and aortic arches are compared for their respective points of origin, tightness of curves, and relationship to other cardiac structures noted in Figures 3-14 and 3-15.

LONG AXIS VENA CAVA VIEW

The vena cava can be identified by placement of the transducer to the right of the fetal spine so that the beam transects the fetus toward the right anterolateral chest wall. This view is important in establishing the presence of normal venous drainage into the right atrium (Fig. 3–17).

SUMMARY

In each view, the right-sided structures (right atrium, right ventricle, tricuspid valve, and pulmonary artery) are compared to the left-sided structures (left atrium, left ventricle, mitral valve, and aorta). The right-sided structures usually appear to be 10–20% larger than the left-sided structures. Table 3–6 summarizes our approach to the fetal cardiac examination.

It is evident to all who do obstetrical sonography that the fetus does not always present itself for optimal scanning of all organs. We have presented the fetus at its best behavior for optimal structure recognition, with the sincere hope that it will aid the examiner in situations less than ideal.

TABLE 3–6. Examinations of the Fetal Heart

1. History from patient/chart (reason for examination)
2. Two-dimensional study of fetus
    Determine fetal lie
3. Four-chamber
    Transverse to fetal spine
    Five-chamber with angulation
4. Long axis/great vessel
    Parallel to fetal spine
5. Short axis/great vessel
6. Arches
    Pulmonary artery/ductus
    Aortic
7. If arrhythmia, or suspect effusion
    M-mode
8. If abnormal anatomy or physiology
    Doppler

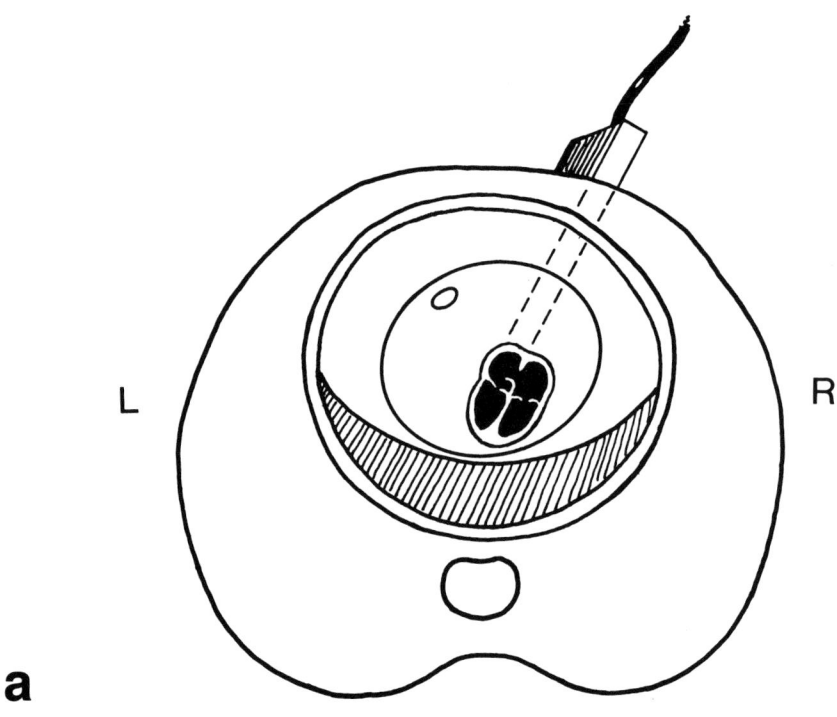

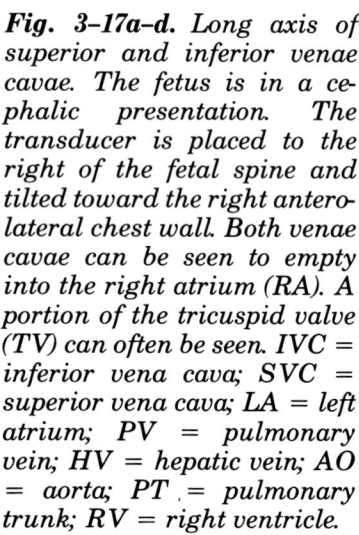

Fig. 3-17a-d. Long axis of superior and inferior venae cavae. The fetus is in a cephalic presentation. The transducer is placed to the right of the fetal spine and tilted toward the right anterolateral chest wall. Both venae cavae can be seen to empty into the right atrium (RA). A portion of the tricuspid valve (TV) can often be seen. IVC = inferior vena cava; SVC = superior vena cava; LA = left atrium; PV = pulmonary vein; HV = hepatic vein; AO = aorta; PT = pulmonary trunk; RV = right ventricle.

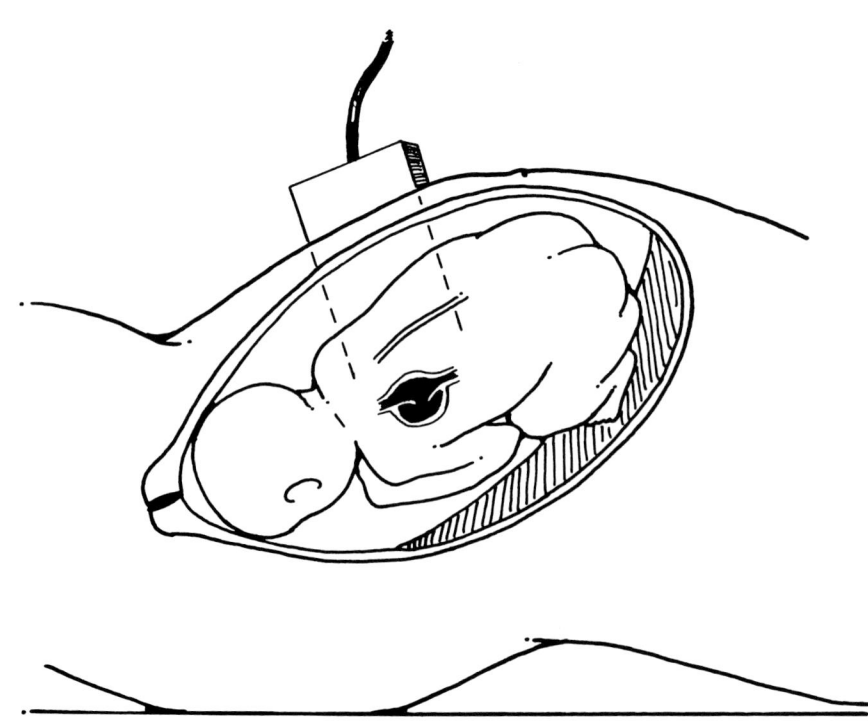

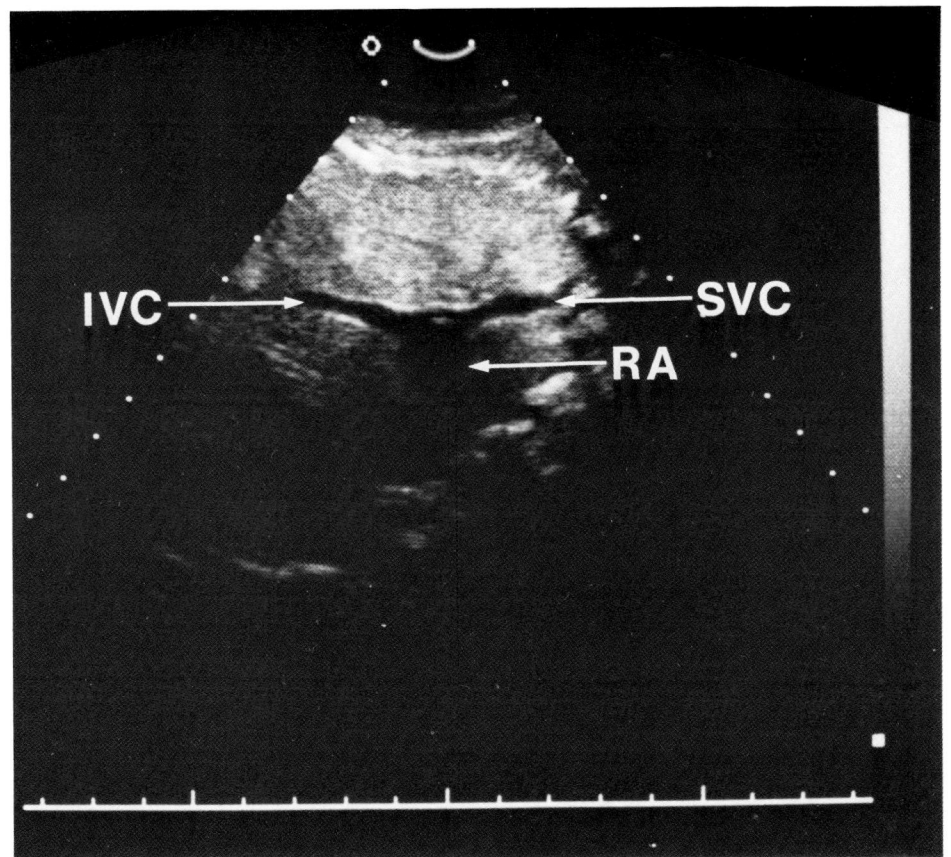

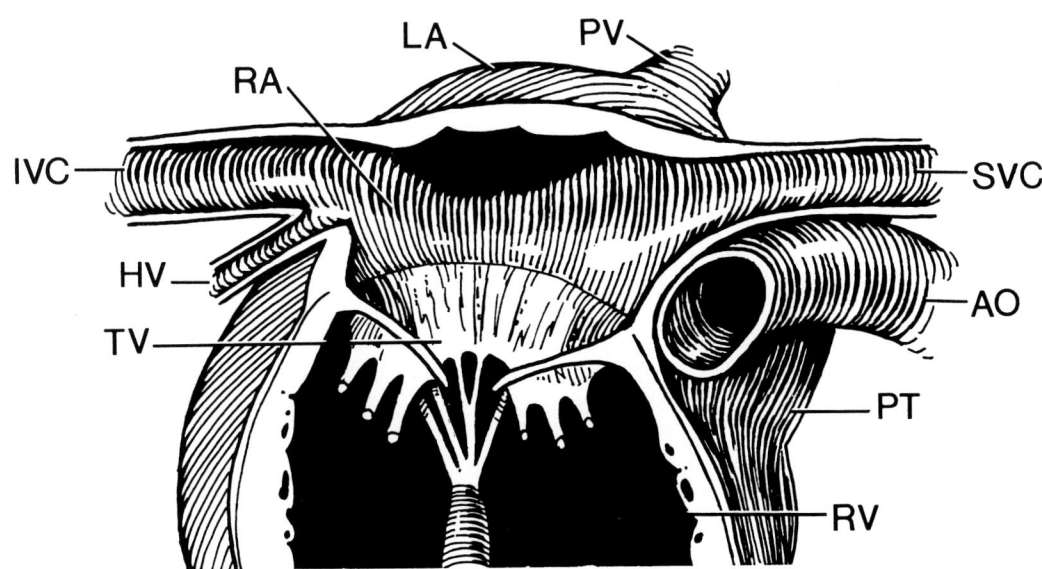

4

The Abnormal Fetal Heart

As skills and equipment for the performance of fetal echocardiography improved, it became apparent that virtually every congenital cardiac defect that can be diagnosed in the infant can be discovered in the fetus.

An abnormal pattern of blood flow through the fetal heart is usually associated with an abnormality of cardiac structure. If obstruction to flow develops, there is often evidence of fluid collection (dilation) proximal to the defect; in addition, cardiac hypertrophy may develop. If the volume of blood flow is increased above normal, the ventricle can also dilate and hypertrophy; pericardial and pleural effusions and ascites may form. As always, the unique blood flow patterns of the fetus must be kept in mind. The ductus arteriosus and foramen ovale are normally patent in the fetus; therefore these problems cannot be "ruled out" in the fetal state. There are reports of fetal compromise associated with premature (in utero) closure of these structures. The blood flow pattern through the fetal heart is in parallel, rather than in series. There is thus some flexibility for the fetus to develop alternative blood flow patterns if there is obstruction on one side of the fetal heart.

The abnormalities found in the fetal heart can be extensive. We have chosen to illustrate some of the more frequently seen types of anomalies.

Performance of a normal fetal cardiac exam requires understanding of normal anatomy. The examination of the abnormal heart requires knowledge not only of normal fetal cardiac anatomy but also of the potential effects an abnormality of the fetal heart will have on other cardiac structures.

VENTRICLES

Hypoplasia

Left ventricular hypoplasia is one of the more commonly seen major congenital cardiac defects. While there have been reports of successful repairs or transplantations, it is generally considered a lethal anomaly. The four-chamber view of the heart appears abnormal, usually with a minimal chamber on the left (Fig. 4–1). Mitral and aortic atresia often accompany the abnormality, and the transverse arch is perfused via the ductus arteriosus. Doppler blood flow velocities should confirm an increase

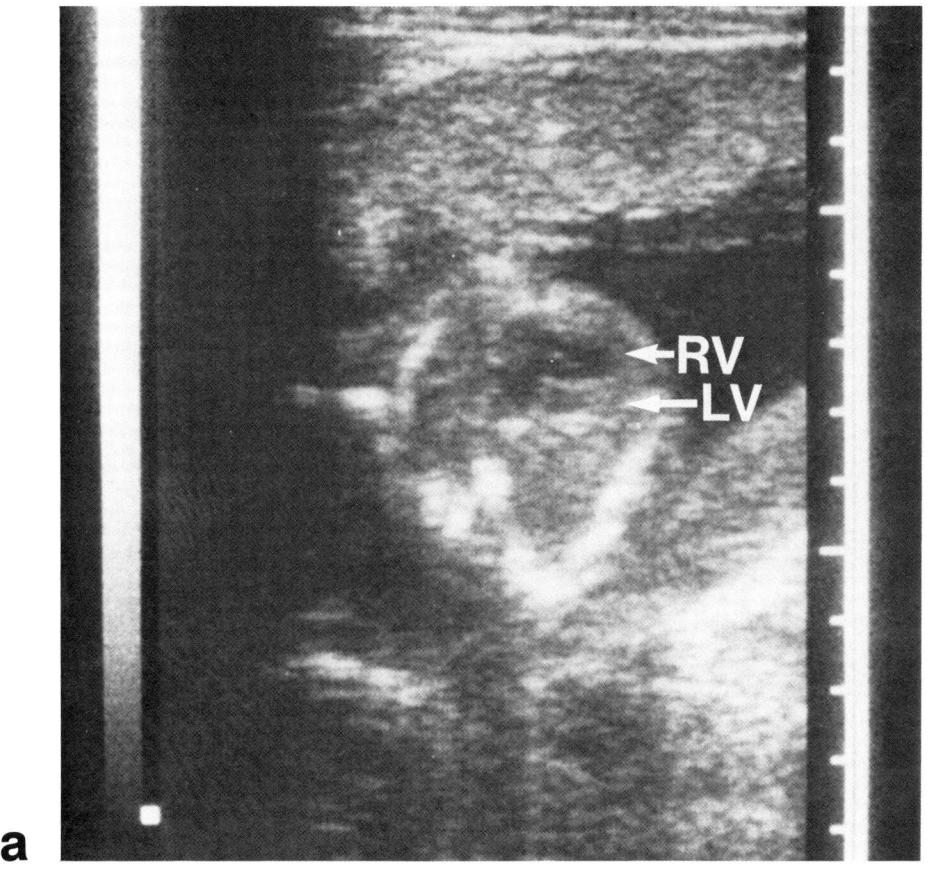

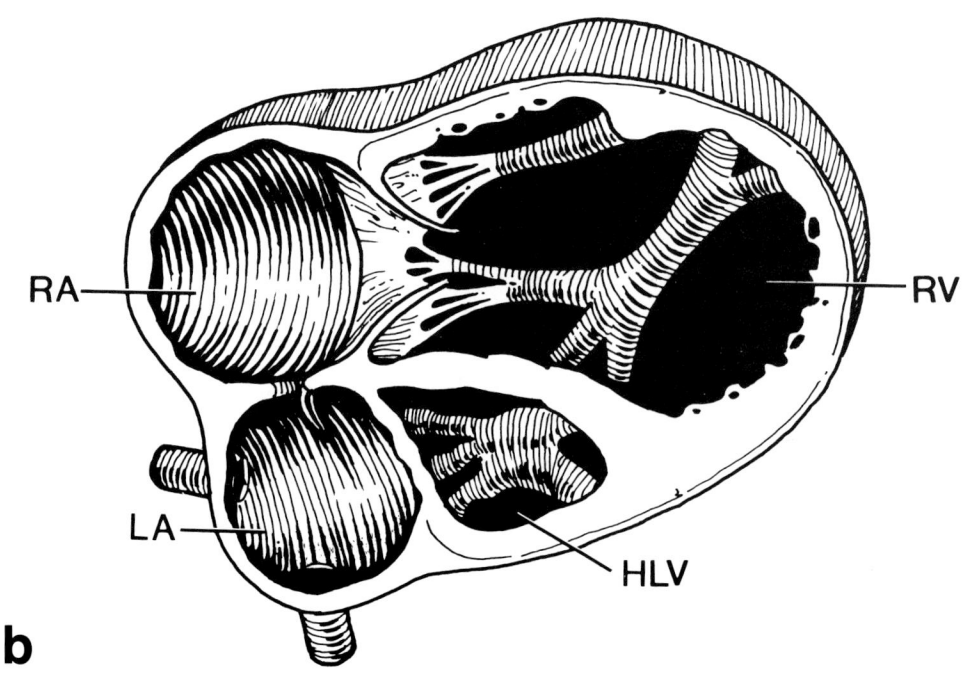

Fig. 4–1a,b. Hypoplastic left heart syndrome. Four-chamber/long axis view of the fetal heart with the fetus in a cephalic presentation and the spine at the 8 o'clock position. The anterior right ventricle (RV) is enlarged, and the left ventricle (LV) is very small. The indications for ultrasound examination were multiple first- and early second-trimester losses and severe asthma. Hypoplastic left heart syndrome can be determined in the early second trimester with careful attention to the four-chamber view. HLV = hypoplastic left ventricle; LA = left atrium; RA = right atrium.

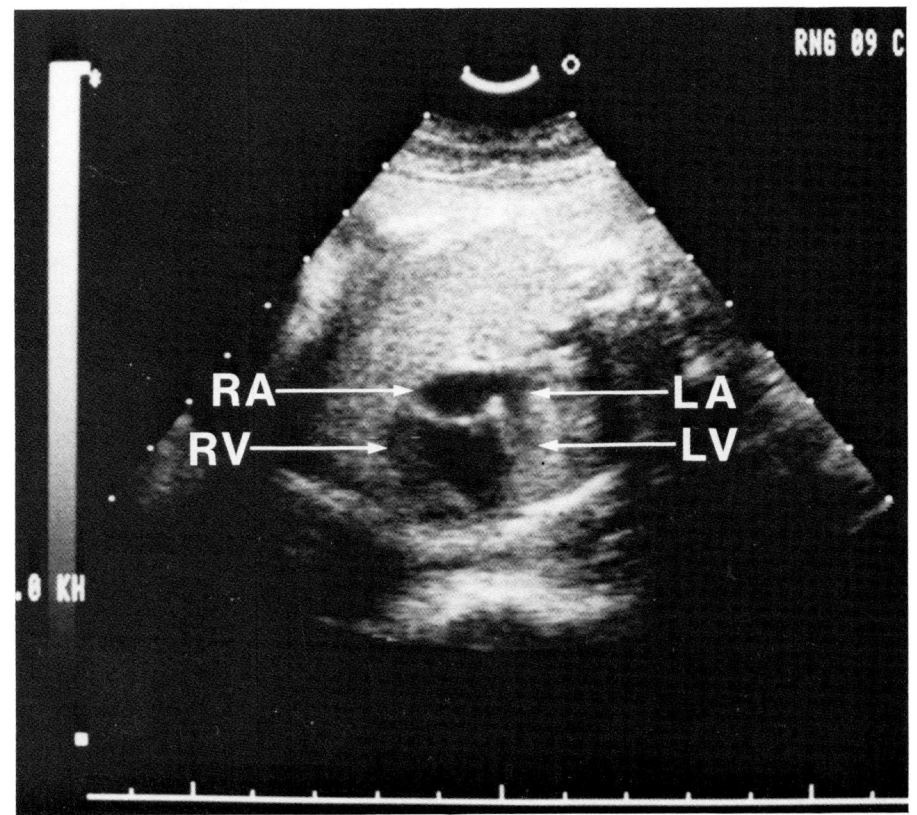

Fig. 4-1c. *Hypoplastic left heart syndrome. Four-chamber view from the base with the fetus in a breech presentation with the spine at the 2 o'clock position. The right ventricular (RV) and right atrium (RA) are markedly enlarged with a thickened right ventricle wall. A very small left ventricle (LV) and left atrium (LA) are seen. No mitral valve leaflet motion could be seen. A fetal anatomical survey was undertaken because the mother has fetal alcohol syndrome and had a previous child with atrial and ventricular septal defects.*

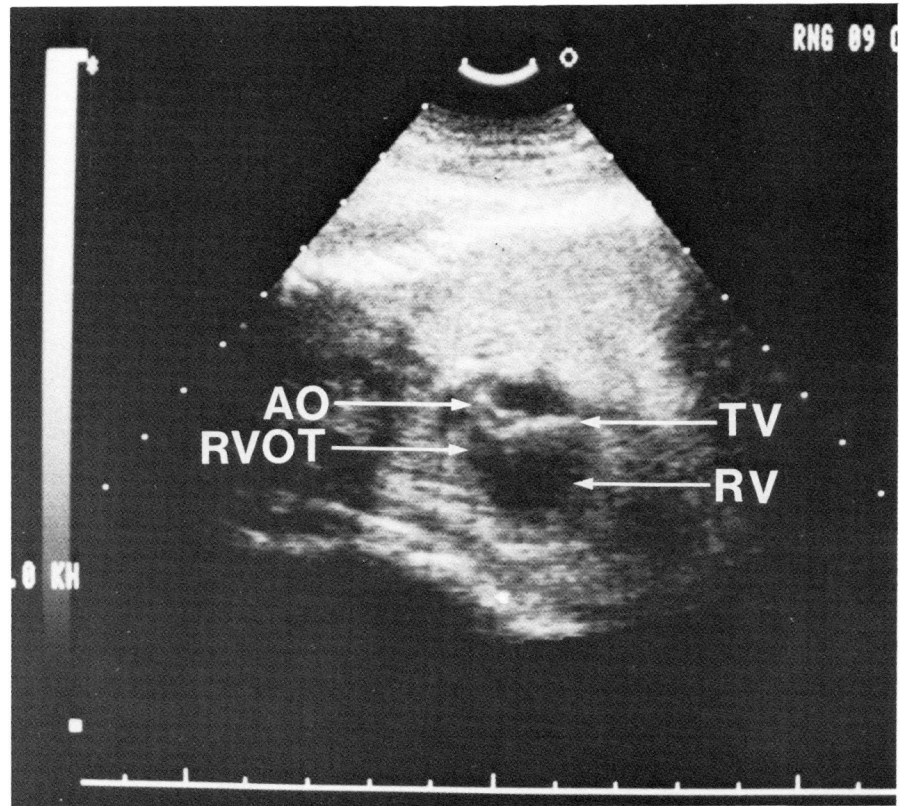

Fig. 4-1d. *Hypoplastic left heart syndrome. Long axis view of the great vessels of the hypoplastic left heart shown in Figure 4-1c. The fetal head is to the left of the image. Medial to the right atrium is a very narrow aortic root and ascending aorta (AO). An enlarged right ventricle (RV) exits via the right ventricular outflow tract (RVOT) as it crosses anterior to the narrowed ascending aorta. TV = tricuspid valve.*

(Figure continues on next page.)

Fig. 4-1e. Hypoplastic left heart syndrome. Short axis view of the great vessels in the hypoplastic heart seen in Figure 4–1c. This view is obtained by tilting the transducer cephalad along the right side of the fetus from the region of the fetal diaphragm. The abnormally narrowed ascending aorta (AO) makes a very small "doughnut hole" with the enlarged pulmonary artery (PA) forming the left border. TV = tricuspid valve.

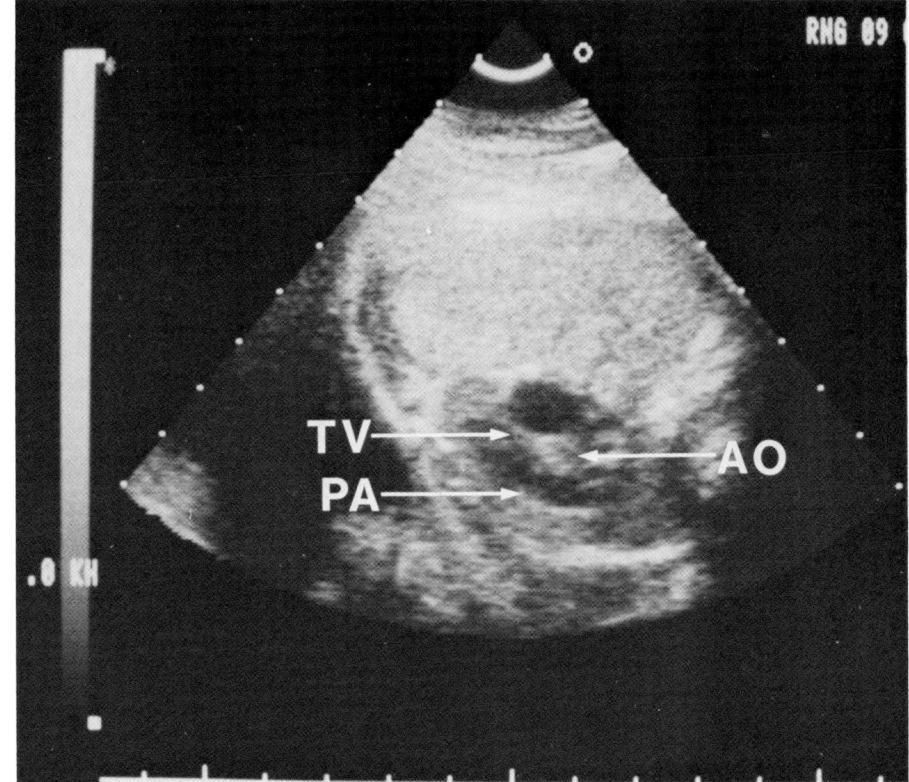

Fig. 4-1f. Hypoplastic left heart syndrome. In this four-chamber/long axis view, the fetus is in a cephalic presentation with the hypoplastic left ventricle (HLV) closest to the spine (at the 2 o'clock position) and transducer. The enlarged right ventricle (RV) again has a thickened wall. This patient was referred because, on auscultation, the fetus was thought to have an arrhythmia. No arrhythmia was noted during cardiac examination.

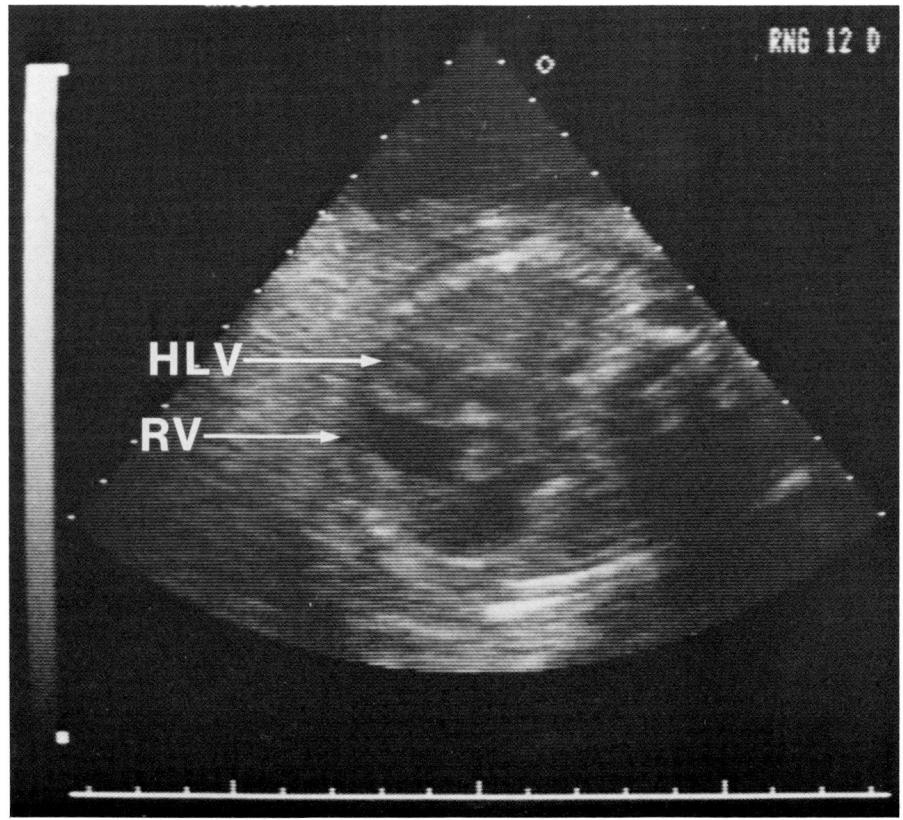

THE ABNORMAL FETAL HEART

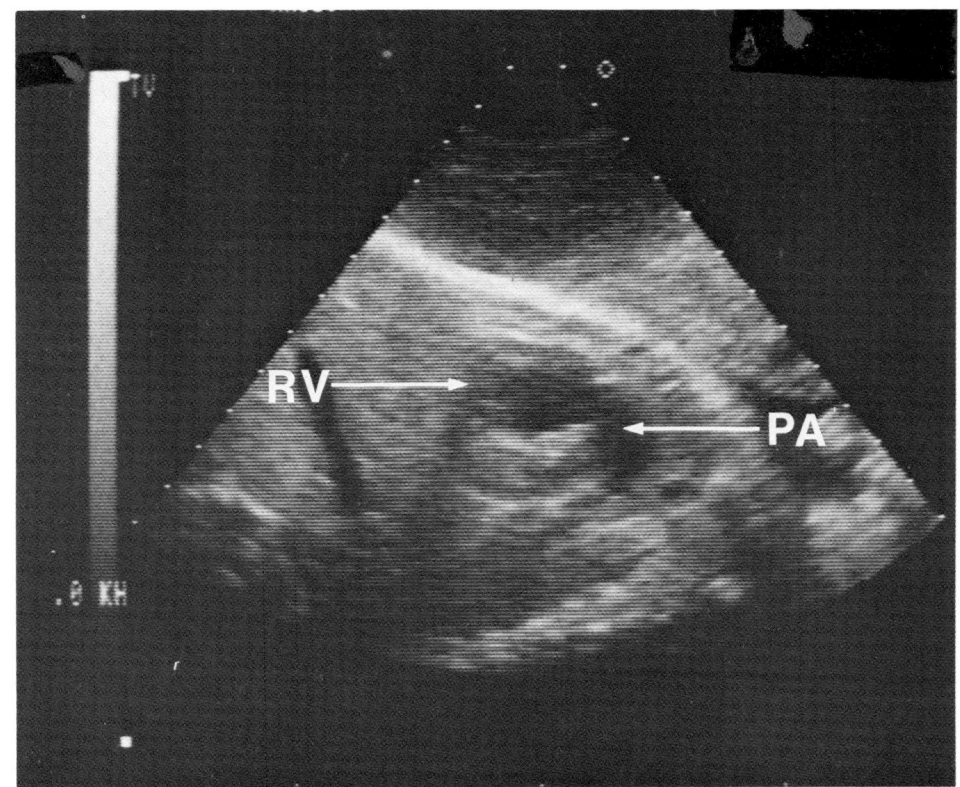

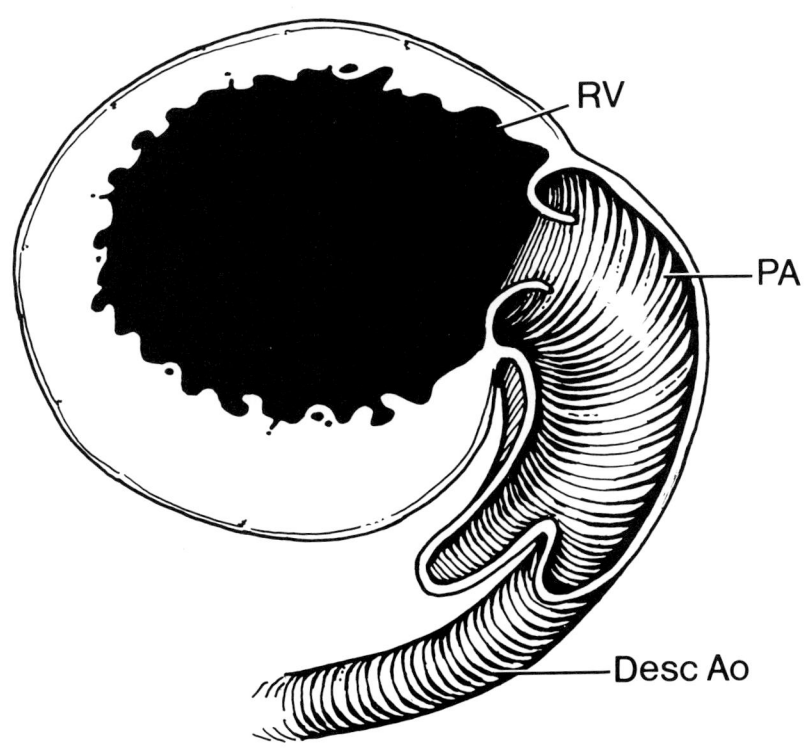

Fig. 4–1g,h. Hypoplastic left heart syndrome. In this view of the heart shown in Figure 4–1f, the fetal head is to the right of the image. This is a cross section through the right ventricle (RV) as it exits through the main pulmonary artery (PA). The wall of the right ventricle is abnormally thickened, and the pulmonary artery is enlarged. Desc Ao = descending aorta.

in blood flow through the tricuspid valve (often with tricuspid insufficiency) and pulmonary artery.

Right heart hypoplasia (Fig. 4-2) may have a similar appearance, but this abnormality has a better prognosis, since the left ventricle, so important for cardiac function after delivery, is intact.

Single Ventricle

A single ventricle may be seen (Fig. 4-3) and occasionally can be confusing if a papillary muscle provides an impression of a ventricular septum. Both great vessels may exit normally.

VALVULAR ATRESIA

Atrioventricular and semilunar valves can be stenotic or atretic. Tricuspid atresia is illustrated (Fig. 4-4). Pulmonary atresia (Fig. 4-5) in the absence of a ventricular septal defect may be a lethal anomaly. The right atrium may dilate, and the tricuspid valve may become insufficient. If the right atrial dilation is severe, pulmonary hypoplasia may develop. Mitral and aortic atresia can be seen with left heart hypoplasia (Fig. 4-1) or independently. The valve appears as a bright echogenic substance, and the leaflets cannot be identified.

VALVULAR REGURGITATION

Regurgitation through cardiac valves can be identified using Doppler echocardiography. This is most often a physiological, rather than an anatomical, diagnosis. Enlarged valves should be examined for the presence of insufficiency. One dramatic example of valvular insufficiency is provided in Ebstein's anomaly (Fig. 4-6), in which one or more leaflets of the tricuspid valve is displaced inferiorly into the right ventricle.

THE ABNORMAL FETAL HEART

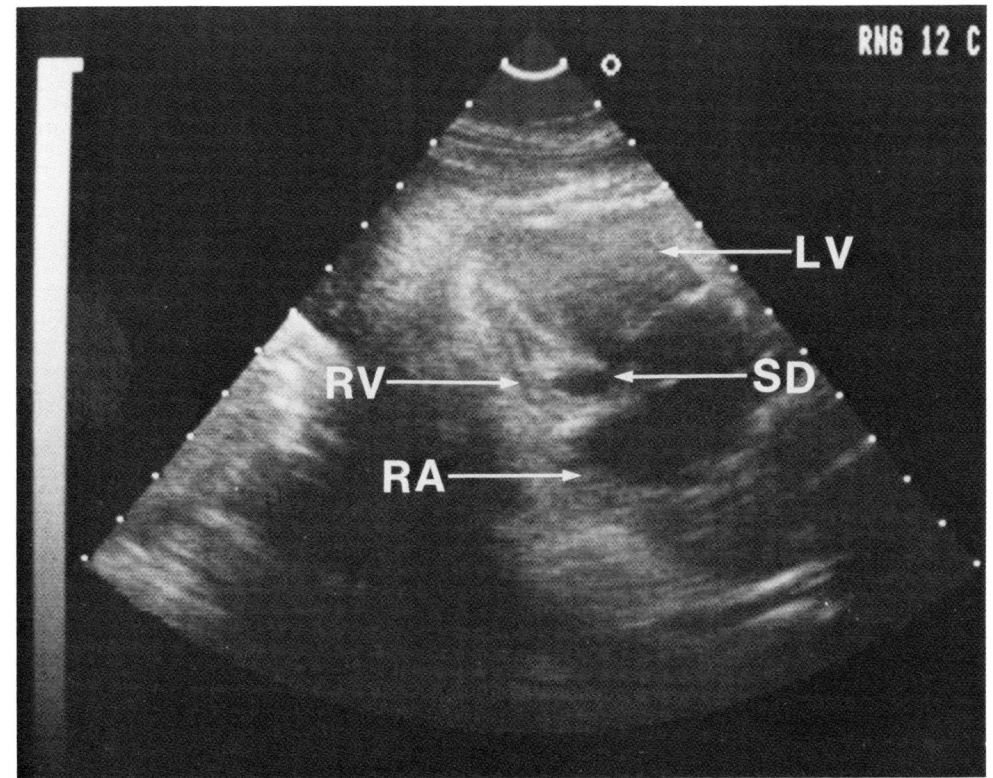

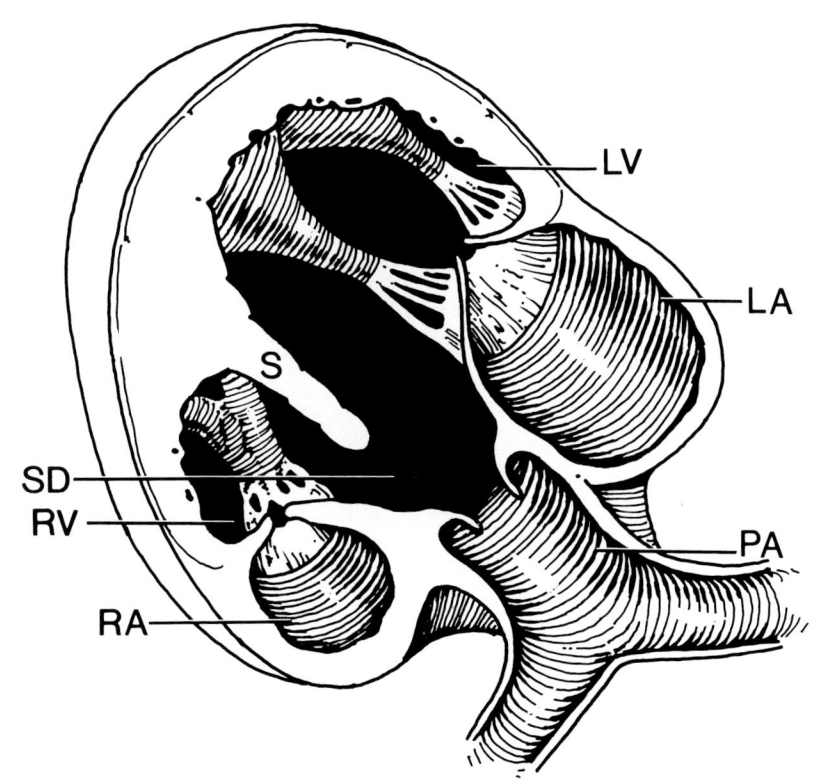

Fig. 4-2a,b. Hypoplastic right heart. In this view, midway between a long axis and an apical four-chamber view, the fetus is in a cephalic presentation with the spine at the 3 o'clock position (spine not in image). The left ventricle (LV) is larger than normal, and the right ventricle (RV) is very small. There is a septal defect (SD) between the right and left ventricles. No tricuspid valve leaflets were seen, resulting in a further diagnosis of tricuspid atresia (see also Fig. 4-4c). Another finding in this patient referred for preterm labor was transposition of the great vessels (Fig. 4-11a,b). RA = right atrium; LA = left atrium; S = septum; PA = pulmonary artery.

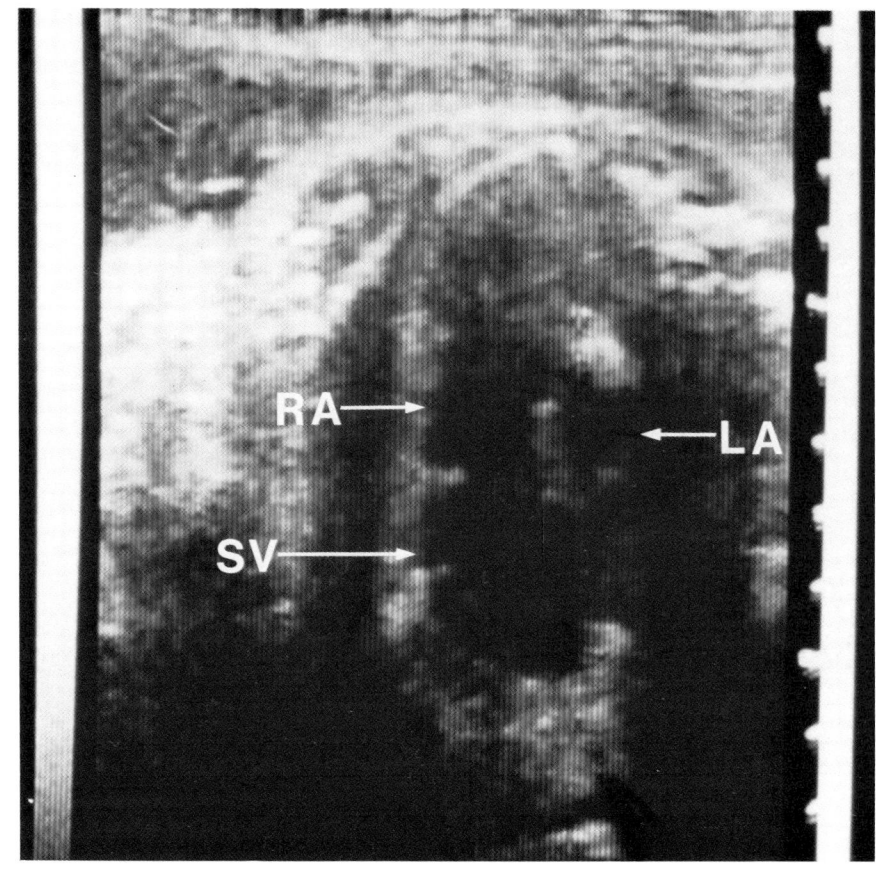

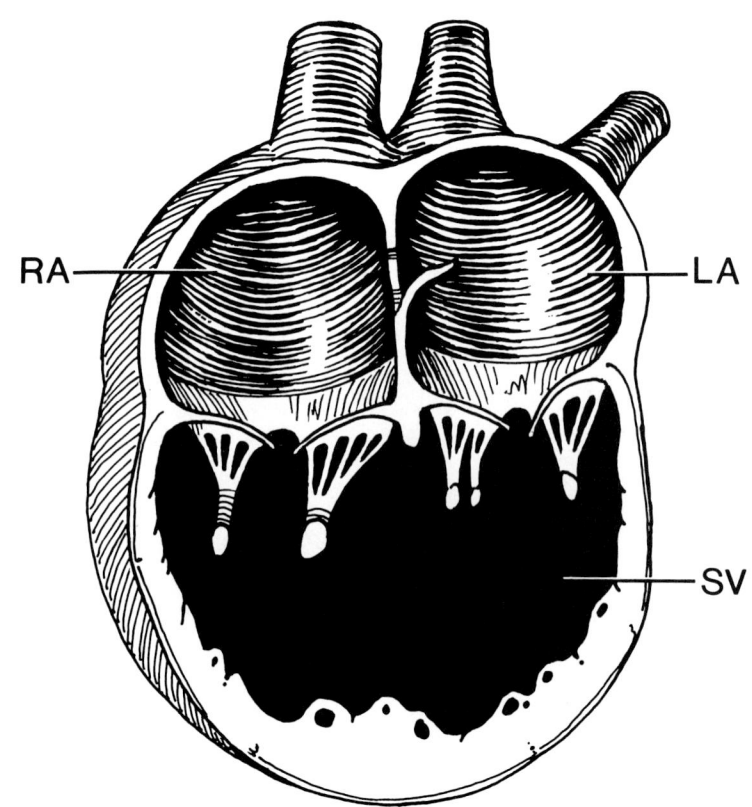

Fig. 4–3a,b. Univentricular heart. This four-chamber view from the base is of a fetus seen in breech position with the spine at the 1 o'clock position. Both right and left atria (RA, LA) are seen with a well-defined atrial septum dividing them. In this view, no ventricular septum could be identified resulting in the diagnosis of a single ventricle (SV). This fetus also had a truncus malformation (Fig. 4–13). The patient was referred because of an abnormal study at another institution.

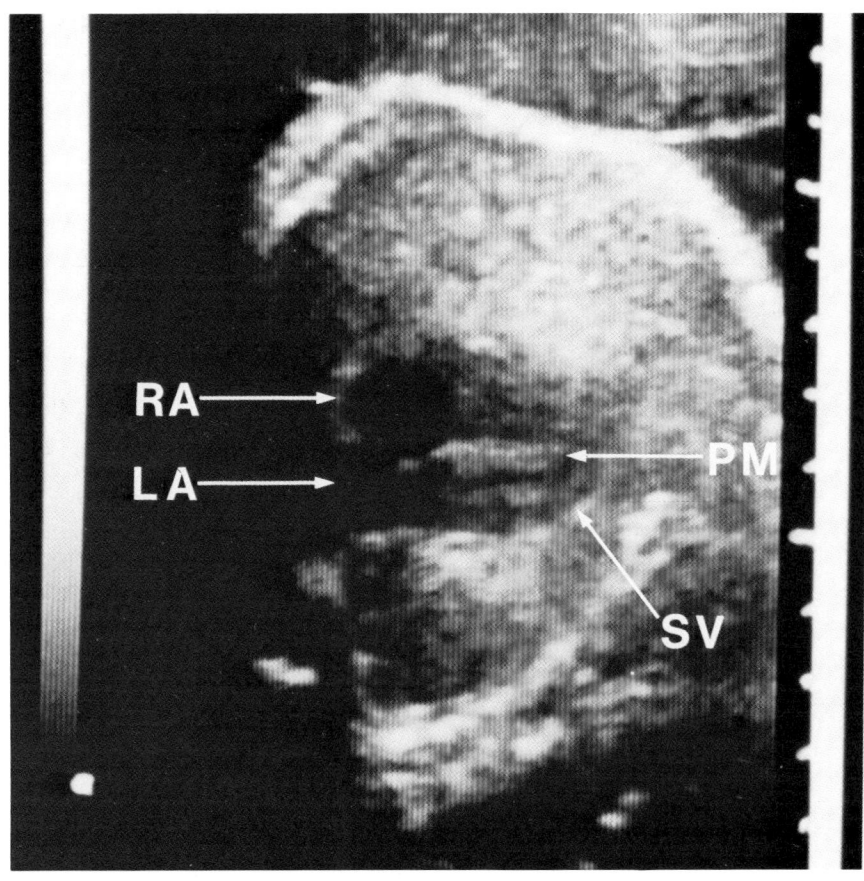

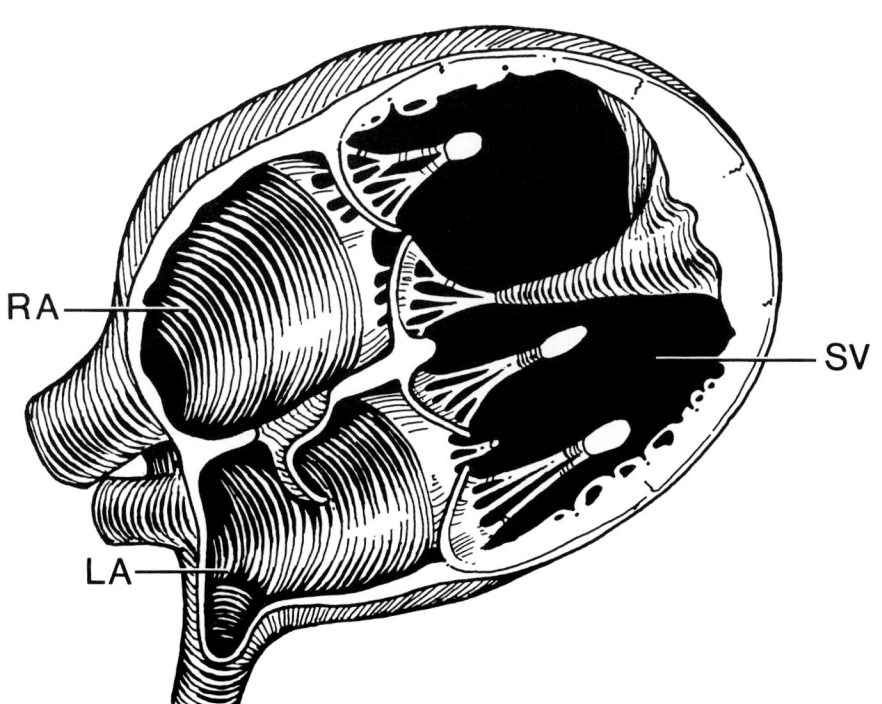

Fig. 4-3c,d. Univentricular heart. This is a four-chamber/long axis view with the right side of the heart toward the transducer. The fetus is in a vertex presentation with the spine at the 7 o'clock position. The right and left atria (RA, LA) are normal in size and position with the foramen ovale flap in the left atrium. In this view, a papillary muscle (PM) could be mistaken for the ventricular septum but was correctly identified on other views (Fig. 4-3a,b). SV = single ventricle.

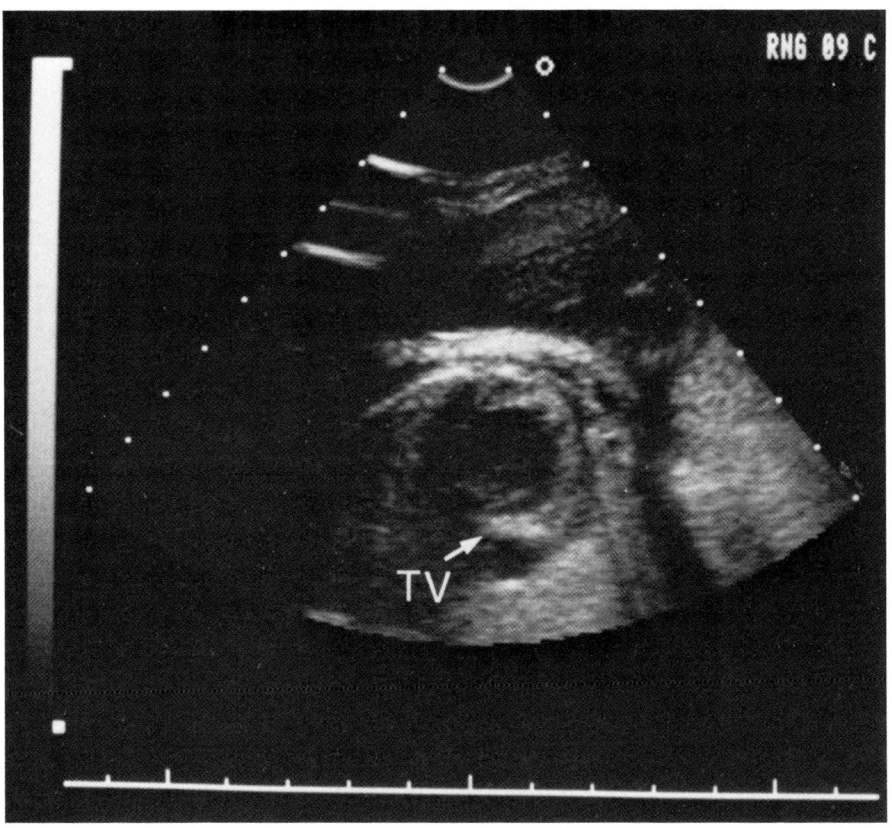

Fig. 4-4a. Tricuspid atresia. In this patient referred for late second-trimester bleeding, the fetus is vertex with the spine at the 8 o'clock position. A large mitral valve was seen at the entrance to an enlarged left ventricle (see Fig. 4-7d,e). There is an echo-dense structure in the position of the tricuspid valve (TV). The single large ventricle has a small inward projection near the right apex. Tricuspid atresia with a large ventricular septal defect was diagnosed.

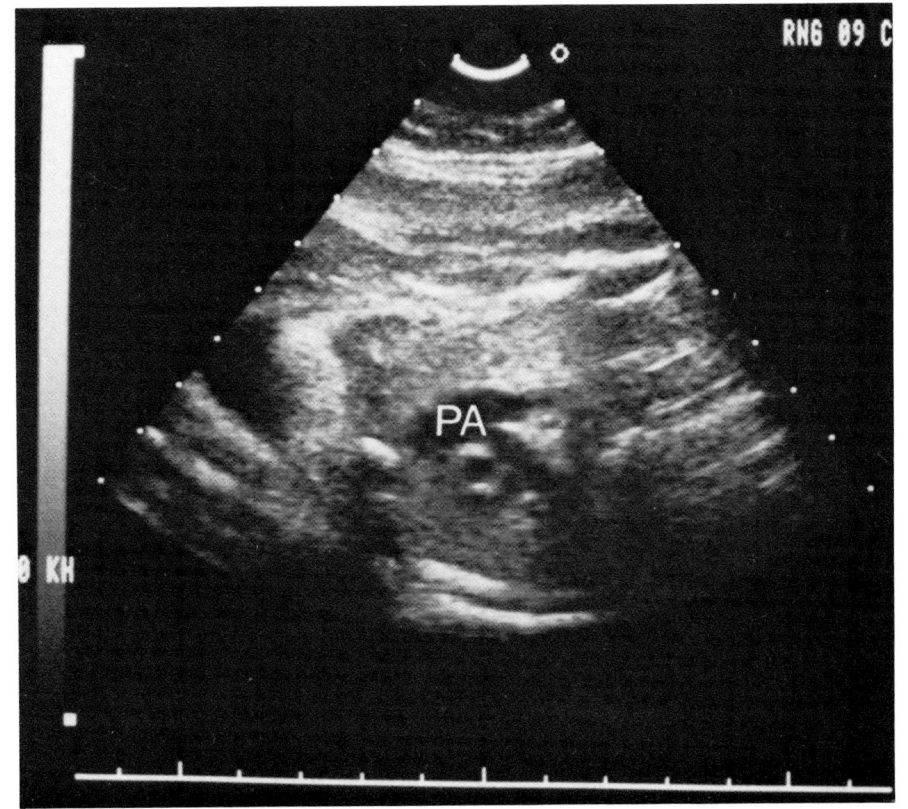

Fig. 4-4b. Tricuspid atresia. In this short axis/great vessel view of the patient referred to in Figure 4-4a, the main pulmonary artery (PA) and right pulmonary artery are larger than normal. At the baby's 6-week postnatal visit to pediatric cardiology, she was noted to have pulmonary artery hypertension and underwent pulmonary artery banding.

(Figure continues on next page.)

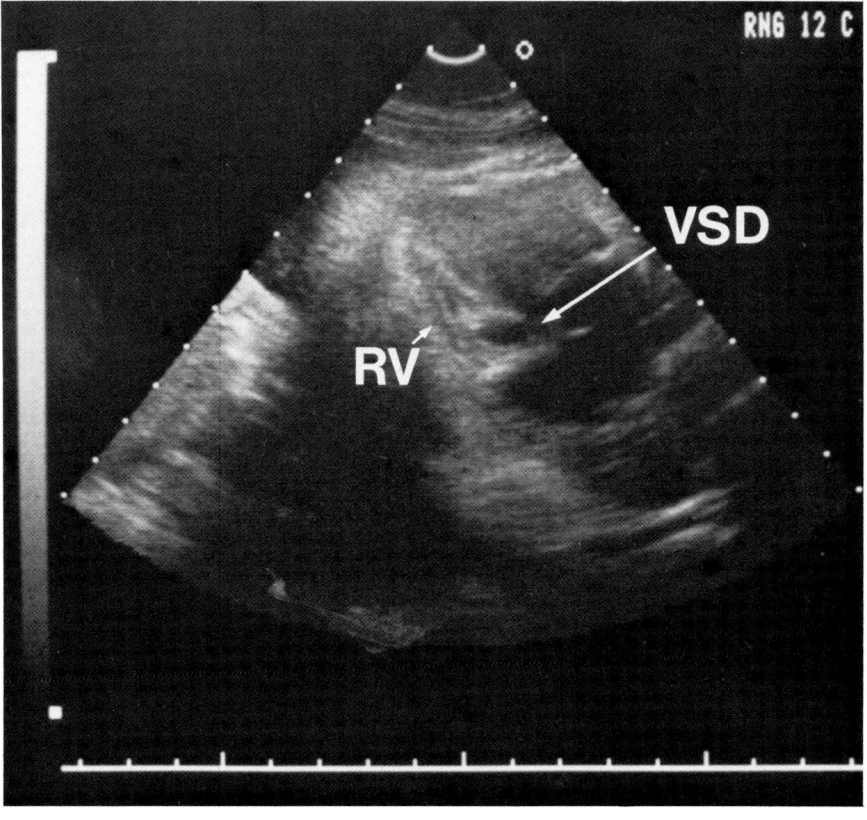

Fig. 4-4c. Tricuspid atresia. In this apical four-chamber view of the patient seen in Figure 4-2a,b, the left ventricle is close to the transducer, with the hypoplastic right ventricle (RV) adjacent. A ventricular septal defect (VSD) is present between the two chambers. An echo-dense band is seen between the right atrium and right ventricle; this band represents the atretic tricuspid valve.

THE ABNORMAL FETAL HEART

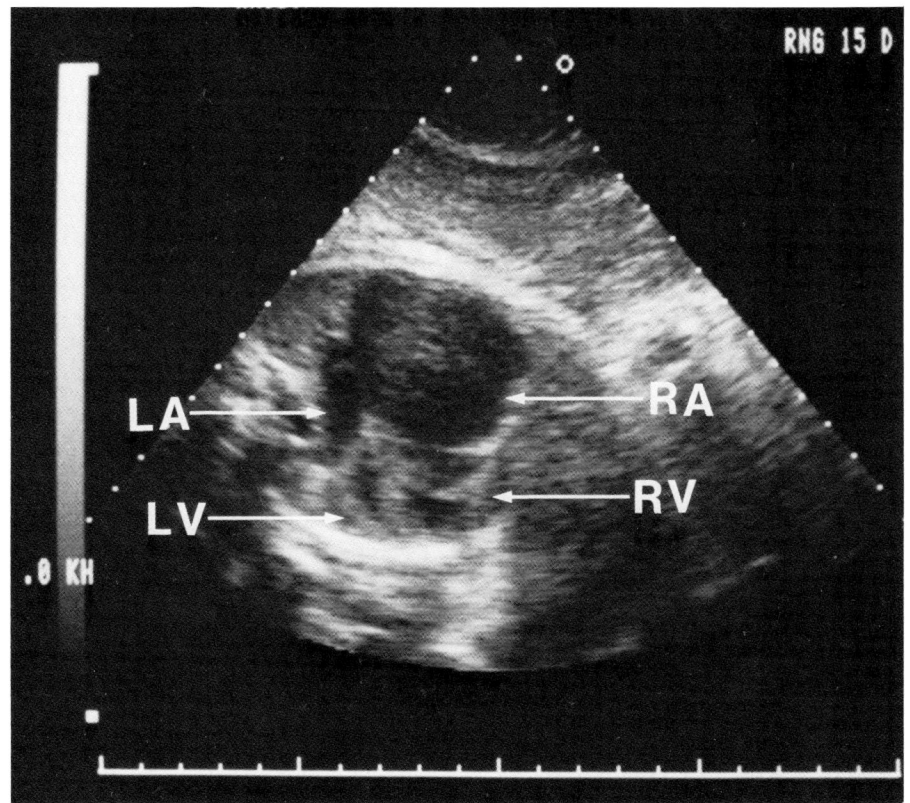

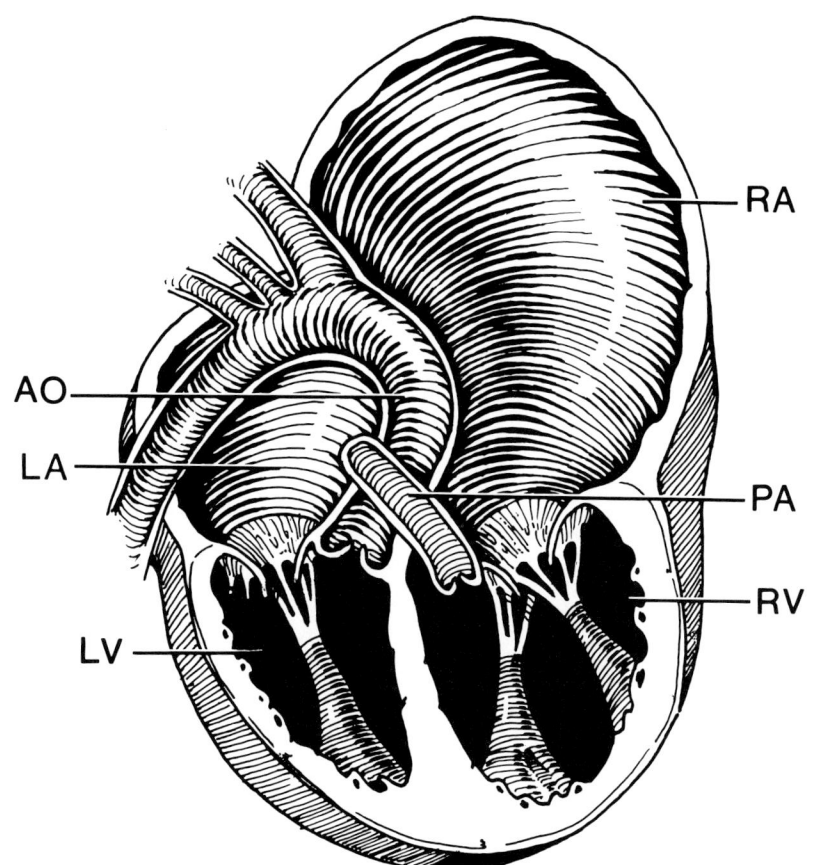

Fig. 4–5a,b. Pulmonary atresia. The fetus is in a cephalic presentation with the spine at the 9 o'clock position. The view is of the four chambers from the base. The right atrium (RA) is markedly enlarged, and the heart fills almost the entire chest. The left atrium (LA) is normal in size but deformed probably by pressure from the enlarged right atrium. The walls of both the left and right ventricles (LV, RV) are thickened. AO = aorta; PA = pulmonary artery.

(Figure continues on next page.)

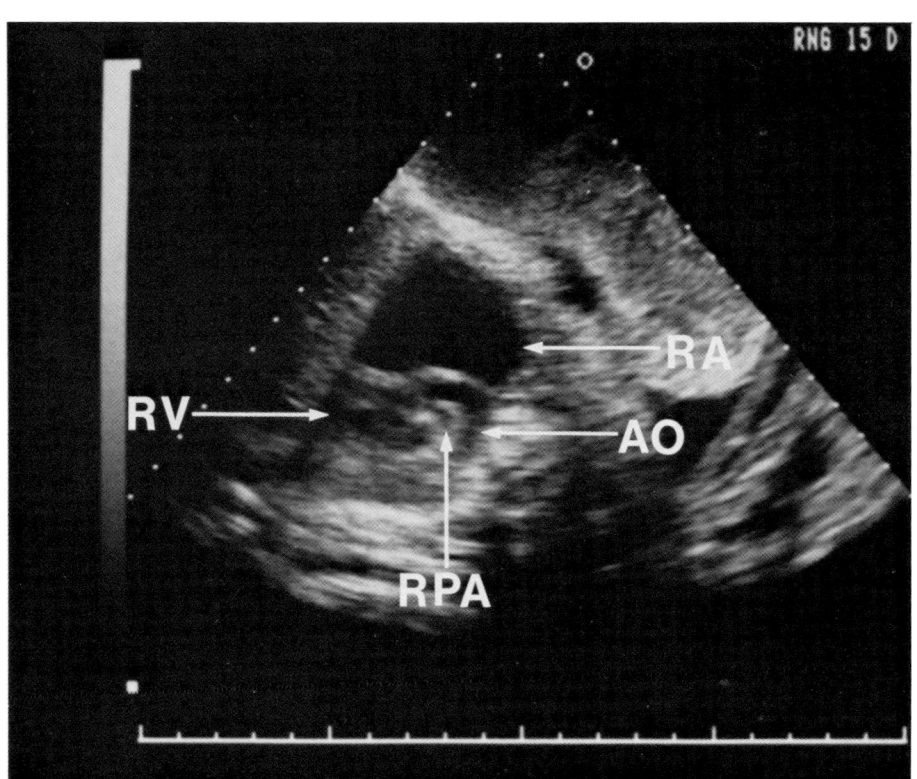

Fig. 4–5c. Pulmonary atresia. In this view of the fetus, seen in Figure 4–5a,b, the head is to the right. The plane is from the anterior portion of the enlarged right atrium (RA) through the ascending aorta (AO) and through a portion of the tricuspid valve and the right ventricle (RV). This long axis view of the great vessels is significant because at no time could the main pulmonary artery be seen exiting from the right ventricle although a cross section of the right pulmonary artery (RPA) was demonstrated.

THE ABNORMAL FETAL HEART

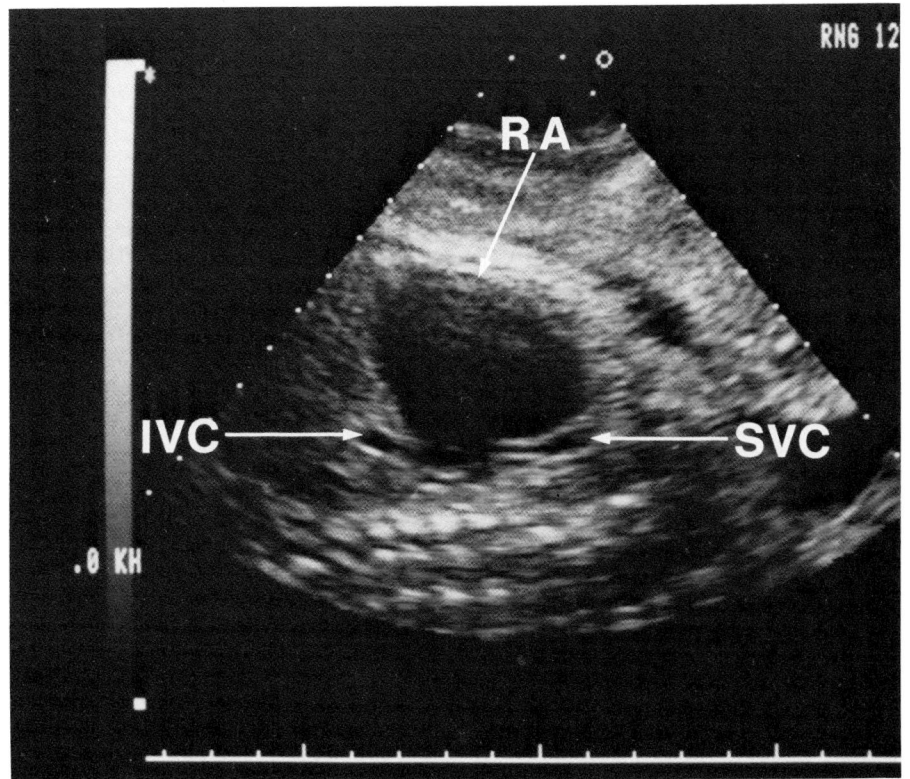

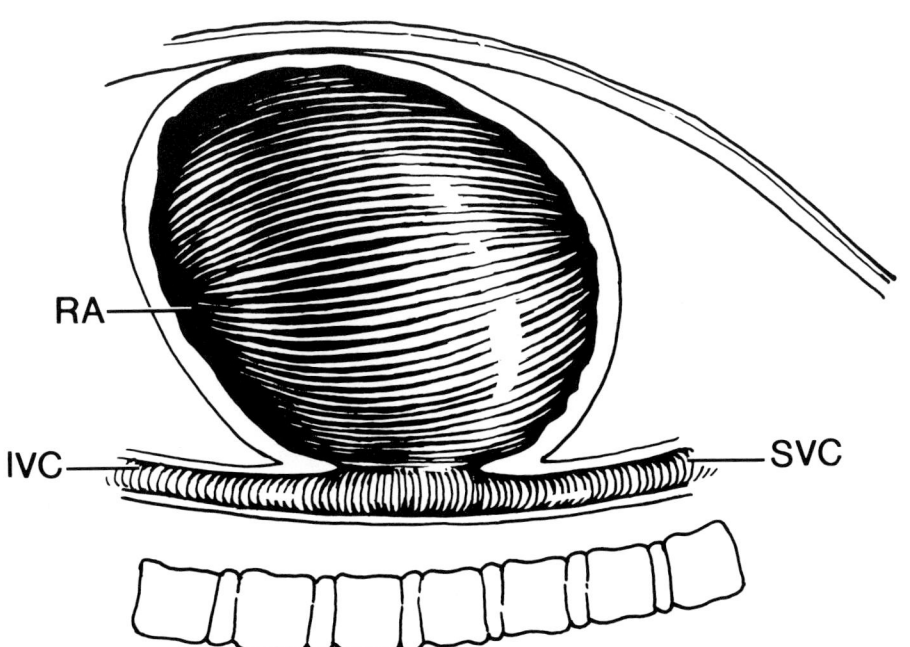

Fig. 4–5d,e. Pulmonary atresia. The inferior and superior venae cavae (IVC, SVC) are seen entering the enlarged right atrium (RA) in this long axis view.

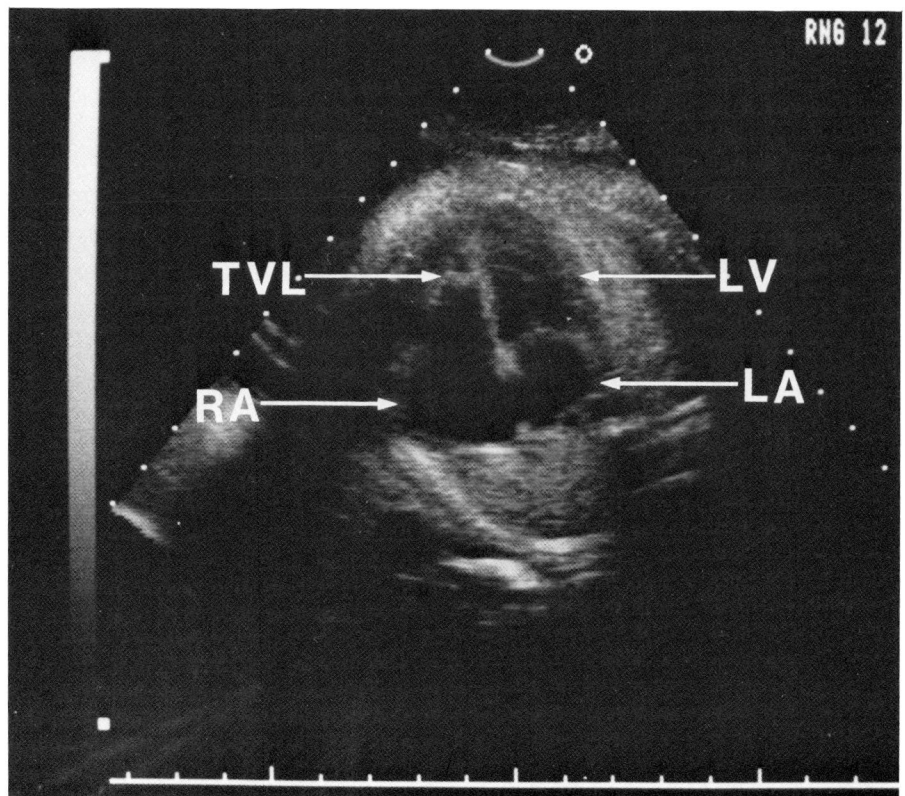

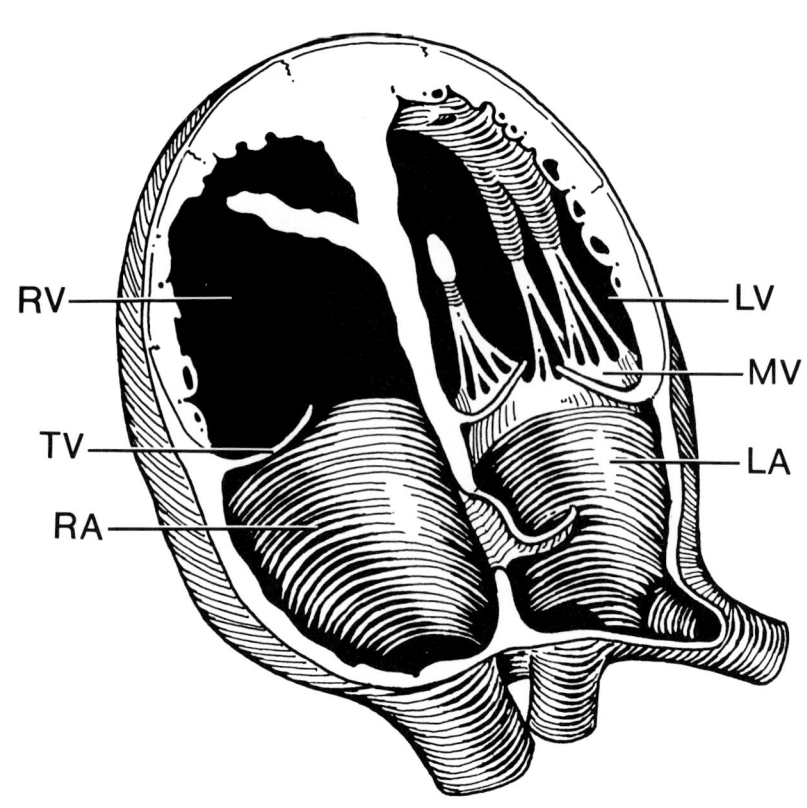

Fig. 4-6a,b. Ebstein's anomaly. This is a four-chamber view from the apex; the fetus is in a cephalic presentation, and the spine is at the 4 o'clock position. The relationship of the left ventricle (LV) to the left atrium (LA) is normal. However, the right ventricle (RV) is atrialized by the malposition of the septal tricuspid valve leaflet (TVL) deep in the right ventricle. Doppler ultrasound studies showed normal left ventricular flows but very turbulent right ventricular flows. RA = right atrium; TV = tricuspid valve; MV = mitral valve.

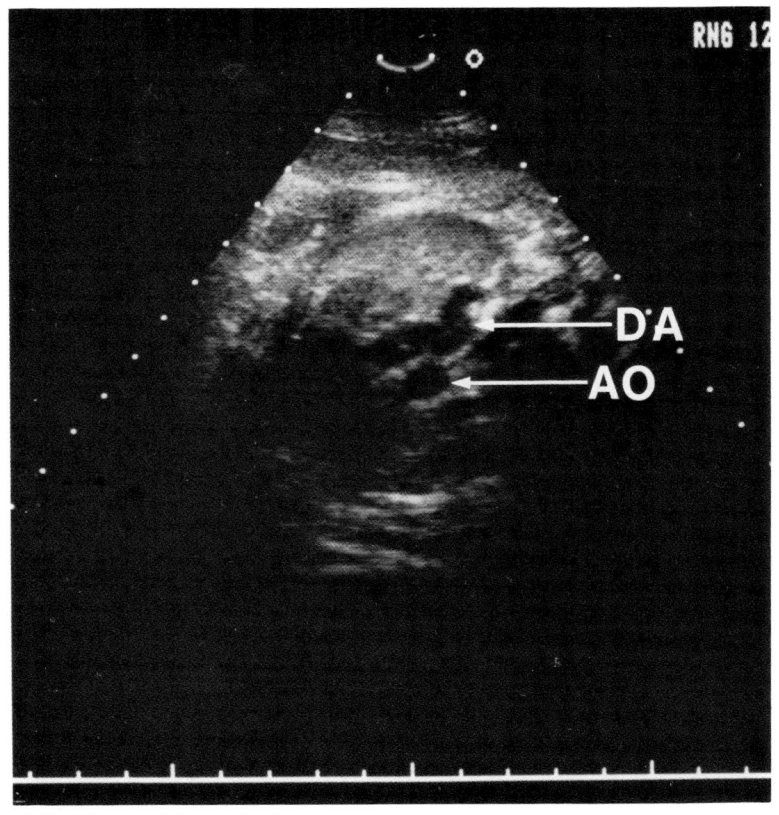

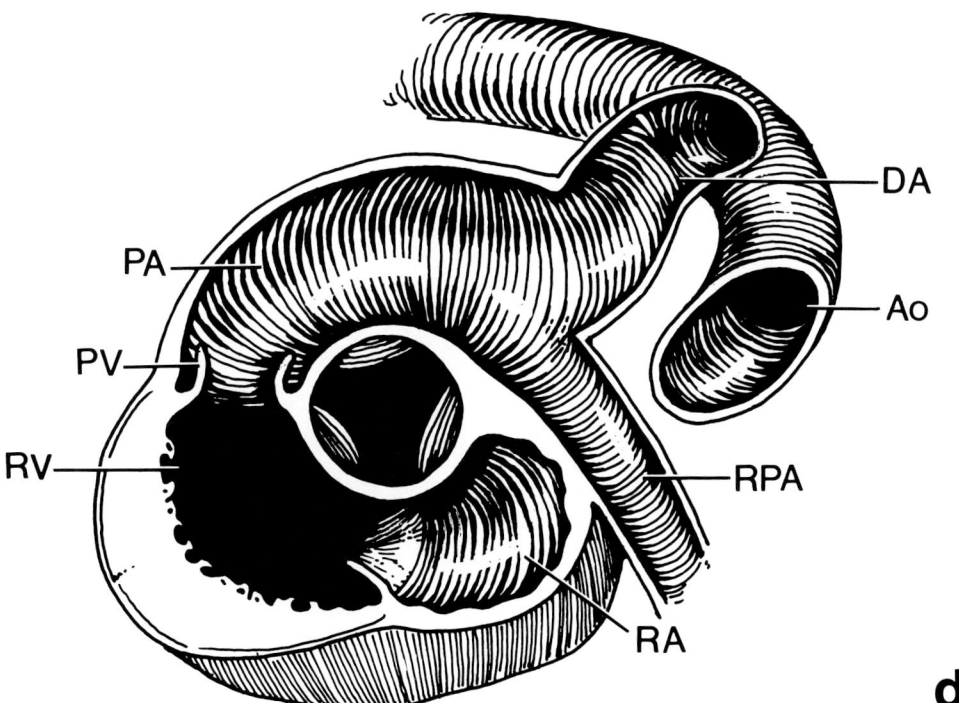

Fig. 4-6c,d. Ebstein's anomaly. The abnormal shape of the pulmonary artery (PA) as it forms the ductus arteriosus (DA) in this short axis view of the great vessels is thought to be related to the turbulence of flow through the pulmonary artery in this fetus from Figure 4-6a,b. The patient had a previous child with coarctation of the aorta. AO = aorta; PV = pulmonary valve; RV = right ventricle; RA = right atrium; RPA = right pulmonary artery.

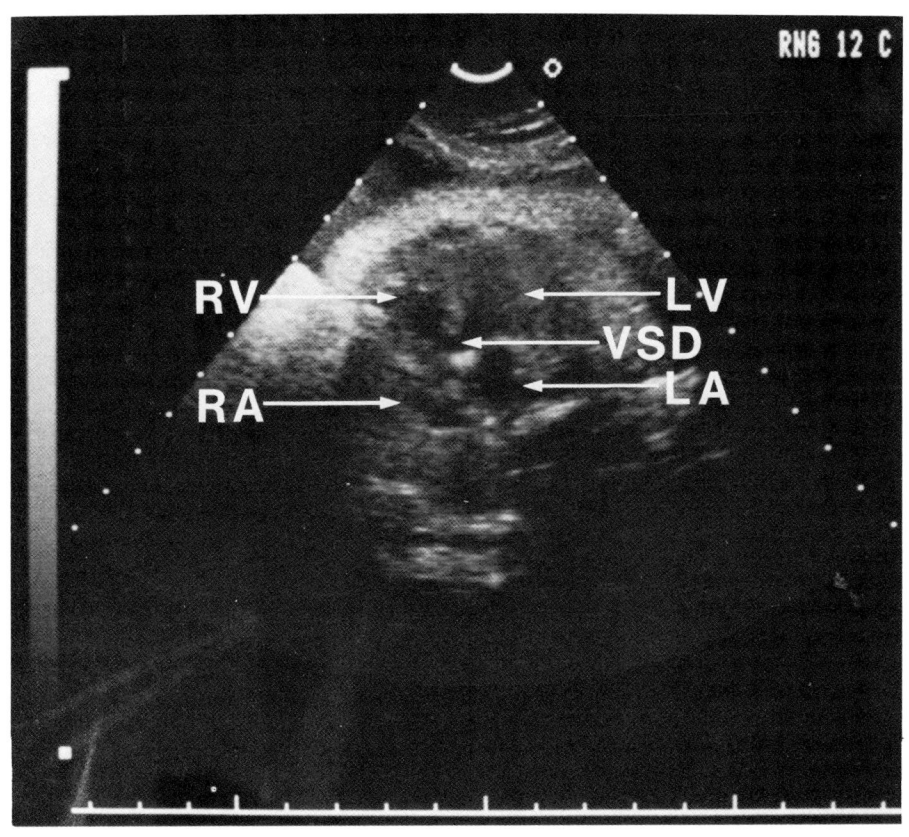

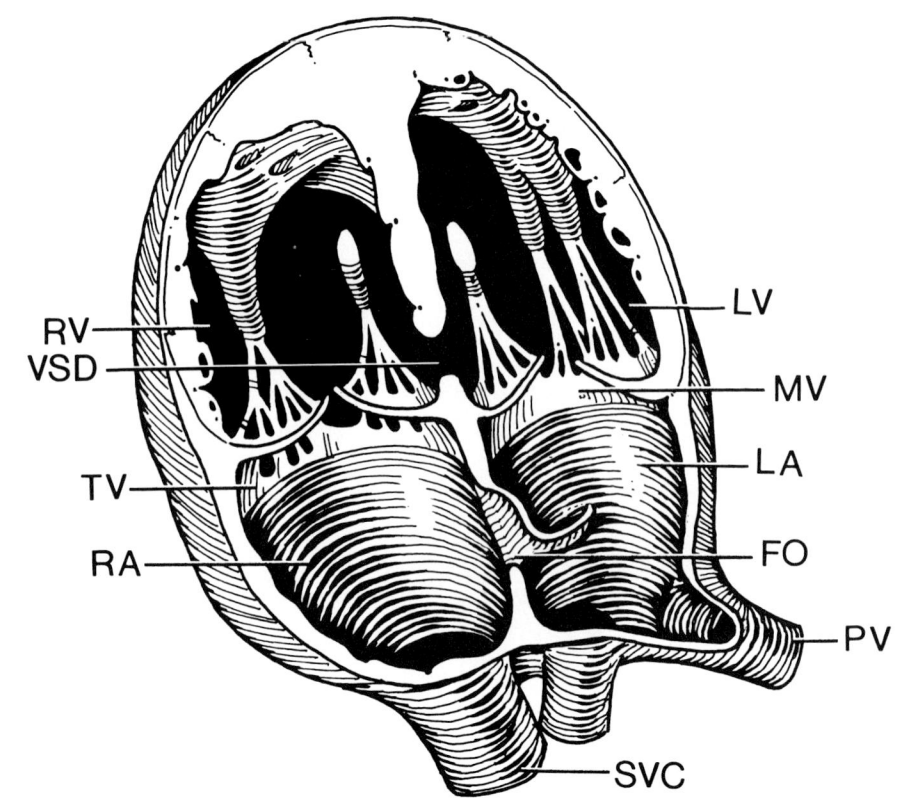

Fig. 4-7a,b. Ventricular septal defect. The ventricular septum in this four-chamber view from the apex is seen to end abruptly about 3 mm from the crux. This small ventricular septal defect (VSD) was only appreciated in this view, which utilized the axial resolution of the sound beam. Cleft palate, omphalocele, and a two-vessel cord were also found in this fetus whose karyotype revealed a 4p- syndrome. RV = right ventricle; LV = left ventricle; RA = right atrium; LA = left atrium; TV = tricuspid valve; MV = mitral valve; FO = foramen ovale; PV = pulmonary vein; SVC = superior vena cava.

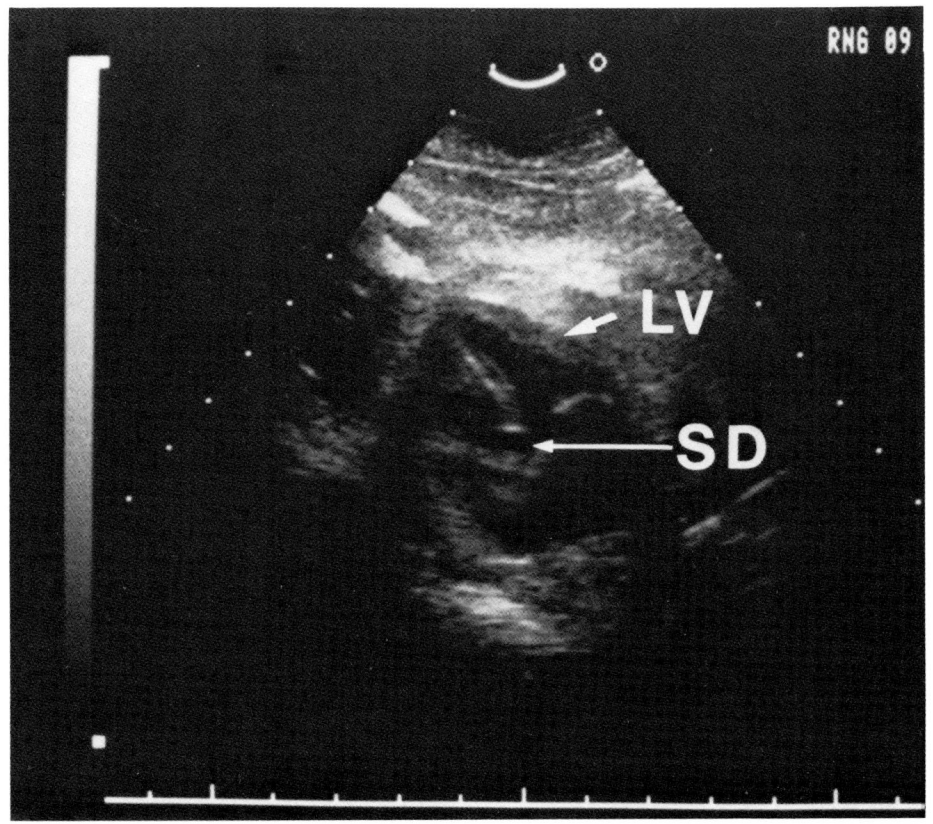

Fig. 4-7c. Ventricular septal defect. A four-chamber view from the apex is seen in this patient who is a class B diabetic. A ventricular septal defect (SD), with normally related and normal-sized ventricular chambers, is present in this view. The aorta was also malpositioned, arising from the right ventricle near the septal defect (Fig. 4-12a,b). An aneurysmal atrial septal defect was also present (Fig. 4-8a). LV = left ventricle.

(Figure continues on next page.)

SEPTAL DEFECTS

Ventricular septal defects are the most frequently seen cardiac abnormality in postnatal life (Fig. 4-7). There are a variety of potential locations for the septal defect. Muscular septal defects are usually lower in the septum. Perimembranous defects are high in the septum. Depending on the size of the defect, these may be difficult to identify. The most easily seen defects occur in the upper septum, and the end of the septum appears as a bright echo.

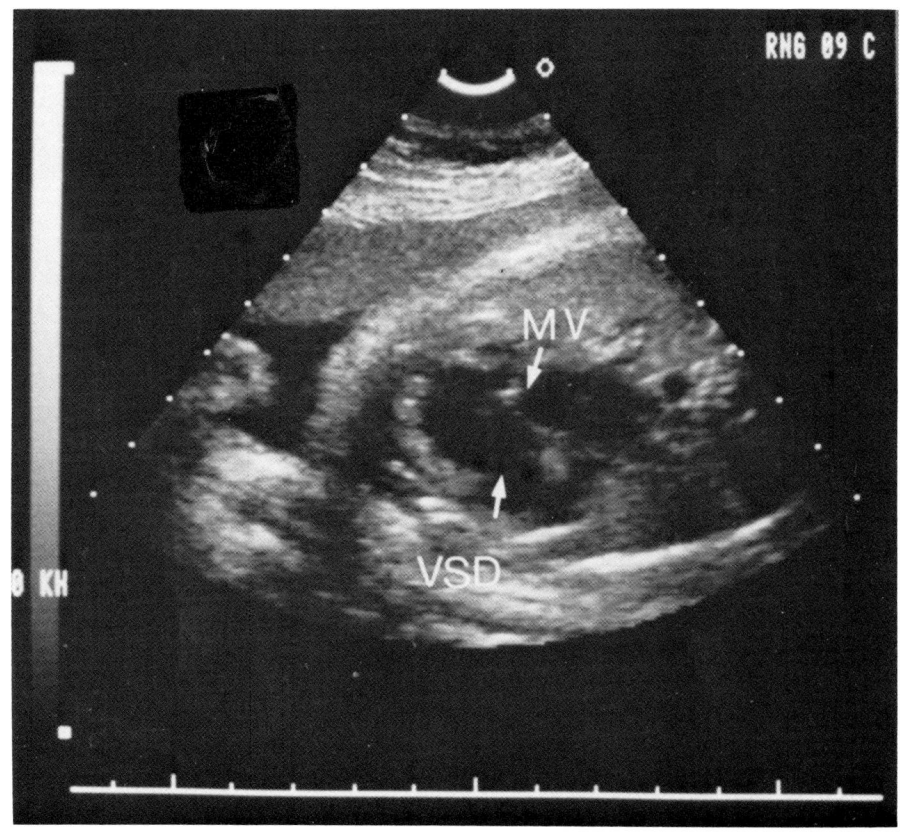

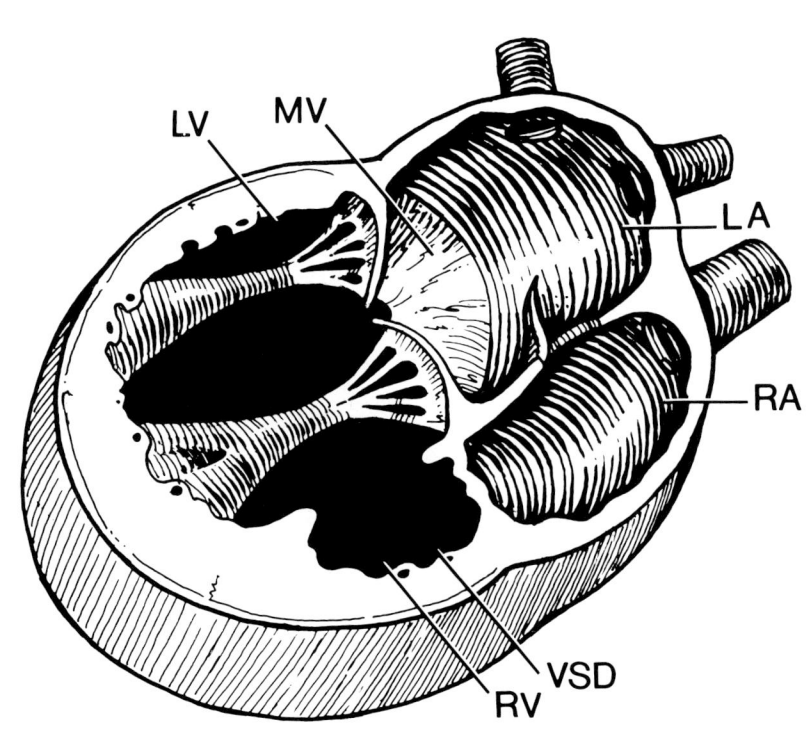

Fig. 4–7d,e. Ventricular septal defect. In this four-chamber/long axis view of a fetus with tricuspid atresia (Fig. 4–4a), the fetus is in a cephalic presentation with the spine at the 2 o'clock position. A large mitral valve (MV) and left ventricle (LV) make up a major portion of the heart. A small indentation along the right apical wall of the heart demarcates the shortened ventricular septum. A large ventricular septal defect (VSD) between the large left ventricle and small right ventricle (RV) is present. LA = left atrium; RA = right atrium.

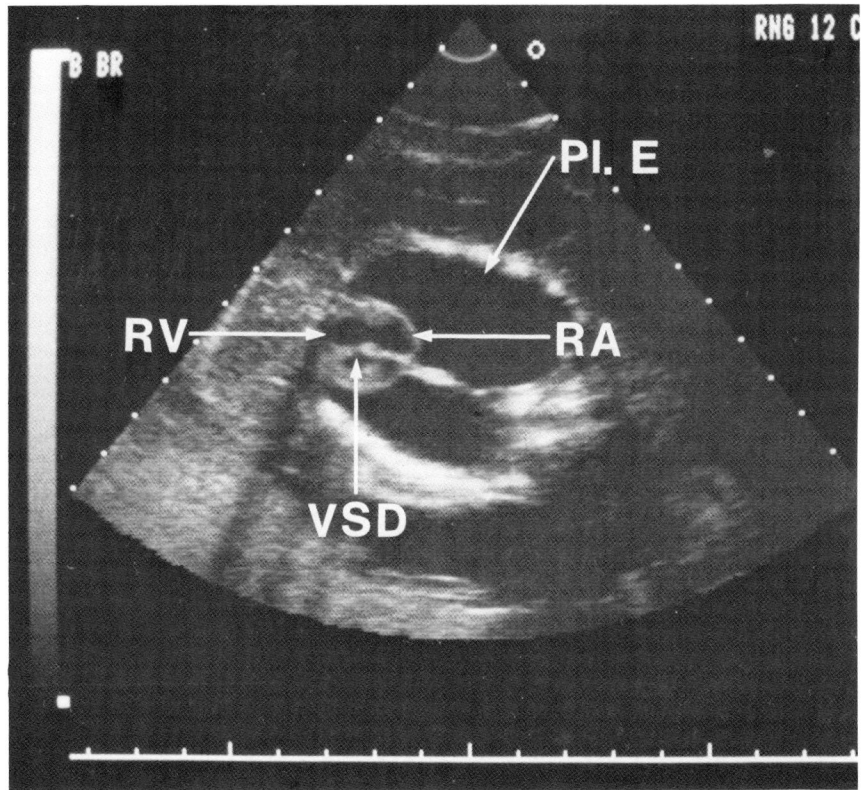

Fig. 4-7f. Ventricular septal defect. This image is of one of a set of twins whose mother was referred because of an abnormal ultrasound study. The heart seen in this four-chamber/long axis view is easily visualized due to a massive pleural effusion (Pl. E). A small break in the ventricular septum (VSD) is seen with some difficulty because of poor lateral resolution. The right ventricle (RV) and right atrium (RA) are enlarged due to cardiac failure. Both fetuses had multiple anomalies.

Atrial septal defects are even more difficult to identify (Fig. 4-8). The foramen ovale is normally patent in the fetus. Absence of the atrial septum (common atrium) can be identified. An ostium secundum defect may also be seen by the alert examiner.

An atrioventricular canal defect appears in a variety of forms (Fig. 4-9). In the absence of other abnormalities, it may may reparable. Down syndrome may be an accompanying feature. The ventricular septum, atrial septum, and atrioventricular valves do not meet centrally.

Atrioventricular canal defect also may be a feature of left atrial or right atrial isomerism. With left atrial isomerism, the inferior vena cava is often not present. Great-vessel abnormalities (stenosis, dilation) may also be seen. In a series of these patients with accompanying complete heart block, fetuses developed ventricular hypertrophy and hydrops. One fetus died in utero, and one neonate died immediately after delivery.

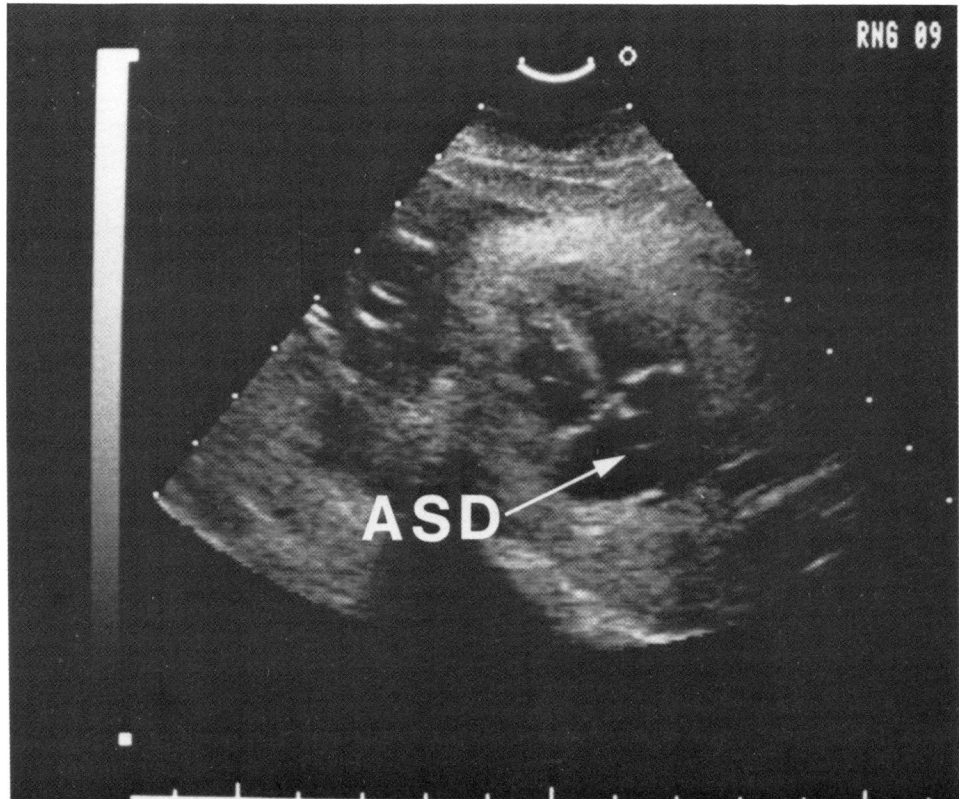

Fig. 4-8a. Atrial septal defect. This apical four-chamber view is slightly caudal to the view of Figure 4-7c. The ventricular septal defect is not apparent here, but the atrial septal defect (ASD) can be seen. (See also Fig. 4-12a,b.)

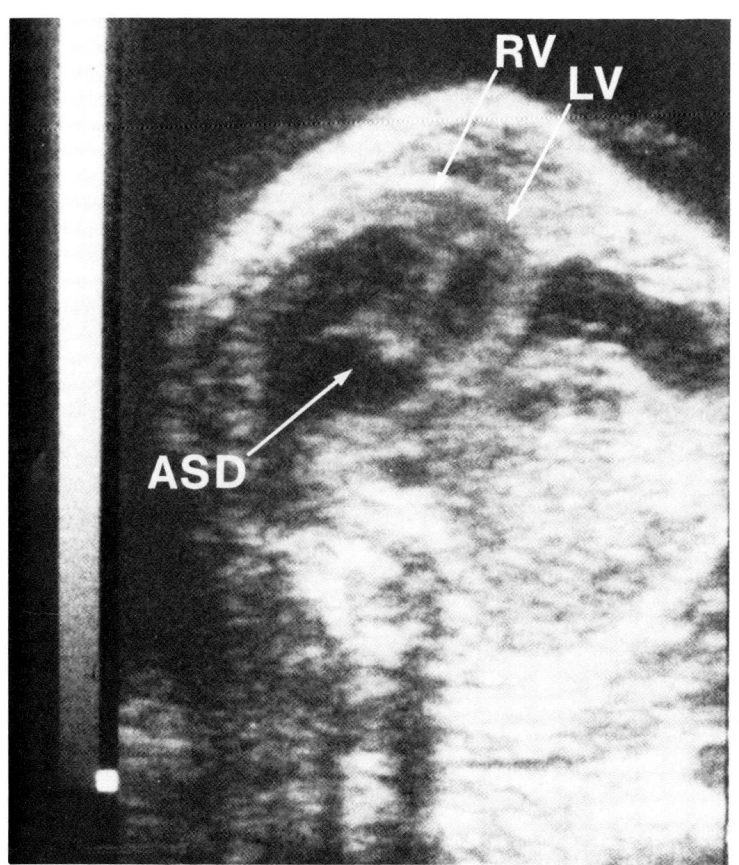

Fig. 4-8b. Atrial septal defect. In this patient examined for size-date inconsistency, the fetus is in a cephalic presentation, with the spine at the 7 o'clock position. The heart is shifted to the right side of the fetal chest by the entrance of abdominal organs into the chest cavity (see Fig. 4-24a,b). A large ostium secundum atrial septal defect (ASD) is present. The heart is otherwise normal. RV = right ventricle; LV = left ventricle.

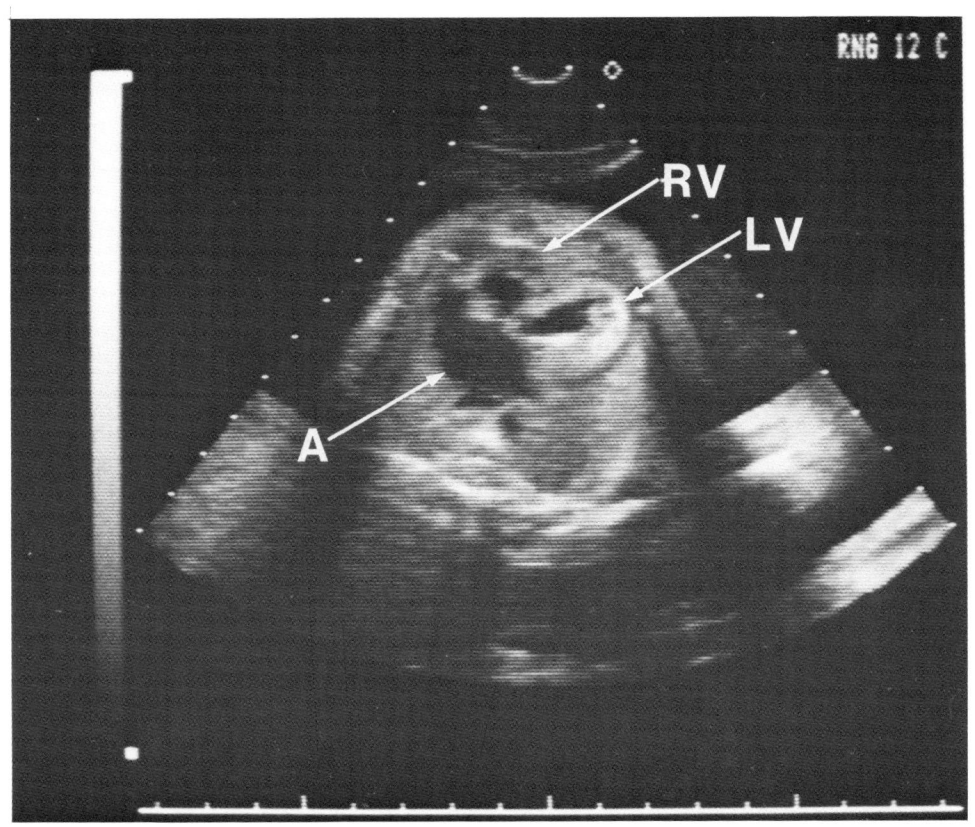

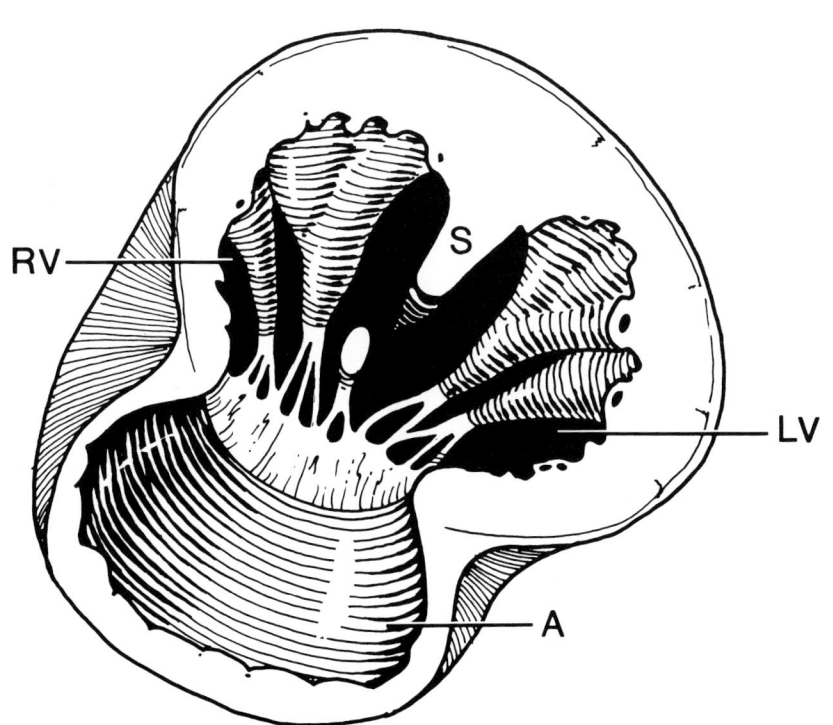

Fig. 4-9a,b. Atrioventricular canal defect. This is a severe example of an atrioventricular canal defect. The fetus is in a cephalic presentation with the spine at the 6 o'clock position. A single atrium (A) is seen anterior and to the right of the spine (image left). Both right and left ventricles (RV, LV) have abnormally thickened walls, and there is a ventricular septal defect and an ostium primum defect of the atrial septum. There is a common atrioventricular valve leaflet. Heart block with left atrial isomerism also was present in this fetus, who was referred for a fetal arrhythmia. Fetal karyotype was normal. (The venae cavae of a fetus with a similar condition are illustrated in Figure 4-16a,b.) S = septum.

(Figure continues on next page.)

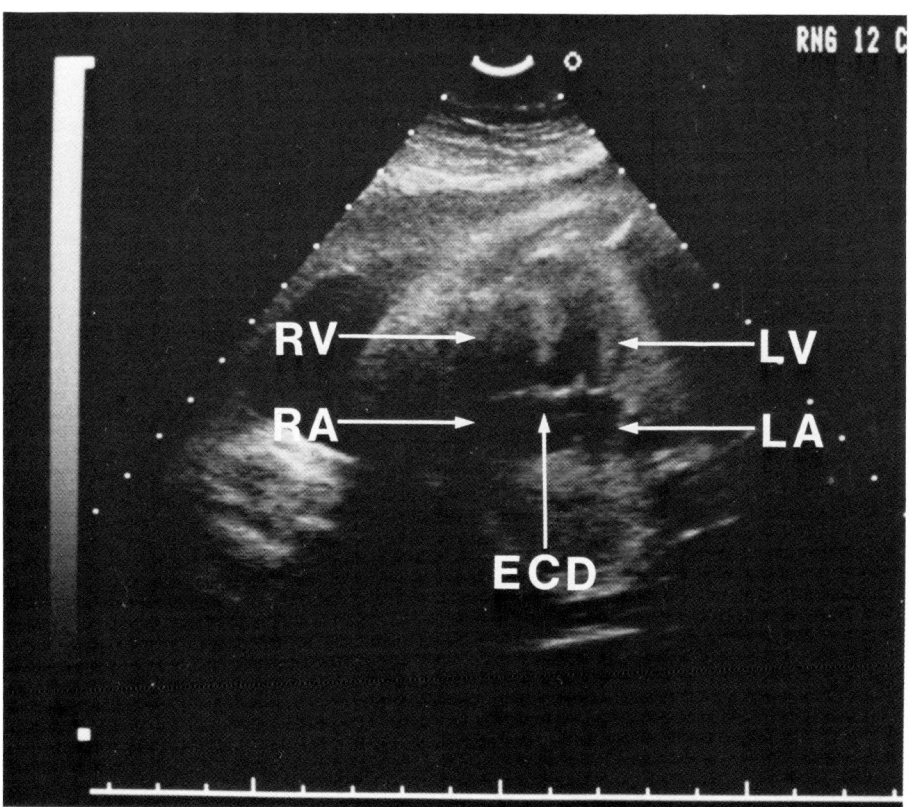

Fig. 4–9c. Atrioventricular canal. Another example of this malformation can be seen in this fetus in a cephalic presentation with an apical four-chamber view. A ventricular septal defect and ostium primum atrial defect combine to form an endocardial cushion defect (ECD). This fetus with trisomy 21 was born to a 39-year-old woman who declined amniocentesis. RV = right ventricle; LV = left ventricle; RA = right atrium; LA = left atrium.

GREAT VESSELS

Tetralogy of Fallot has been identified in the fetus (Fig. 4–10). The features are usually restricted to the overriding aorta and ventricular septal defect. Pulmonary atresia may become more apparent as the pregnancy progresses. Right ventricular hypertrophy may not develop prior to delivery. Because tetralogy of Fallot is frequently seen in the fetus with Down syndrome, karyotyping should be considered.

Transposition of the great vessels (Fig. 4–11) comes in two major varieties. In the one most commonly seen, the aorta is connected to the "right" (anterior) ventricle, and the pulmonary artery exits from the "left" (posterior) ventricle. It is also possible for the great vessels to be in the normal position, along with the venae cavae and pulmonary veins, but with the ventricles are reversed ("corrected transposition"). Careful attention to the arch studies will help to identify uncorrected transposition. Since both great vessels may have an "arch" appearance, the aorta is identified as the one with the vessels exiting into the head. Unless this determination is made, transposition is not ruled out.

Double-outlet right ventricle occurs when both great vessels exit from the same (right) ventricle (Fig. 4–12).

Truncus arteriosus occurs when incomplete separation of the great vessels is present (Fig. 4–13). A variety of patterns is possible.

Coarctation of the aorta may be difficult to identify in the fetus. A shift in anatomy with the postnatal closure of the ductus may result in a coarctation becoming apparent. In fetal life, if there is a disproportionate enlargement of the right ventricle, an interruption of the aortic arch (Fig. 4–14) or coarctation of the aorta (Fig. 4–15) should be considered. Since the left ventricular blood flow is restricted, an increase in blood flow occurs through the right ventricle.

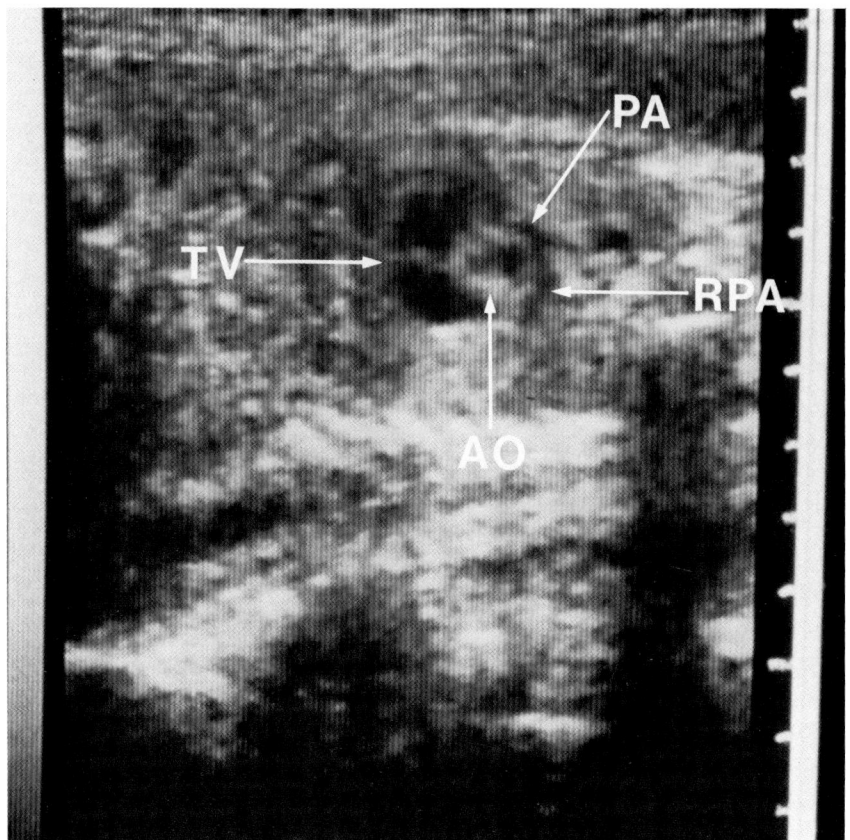

Fig. 4–10a,b. Tetralogy of Fallot. In this short axis view of the great vessels, the anterior right ventricle (RV) exits through a severely narrowed pulmonary artery (PA), which wraps around an enlarged ascending aorta (AO). The patient had a previous child with tetralogy of Fallot who was otherwise normal. This fetus, however, was found at birth to have trisomy 21. RPA = right pulmonary artery; TV = tricuspid valve; PV = pulmonary valve; RA = right atrium.

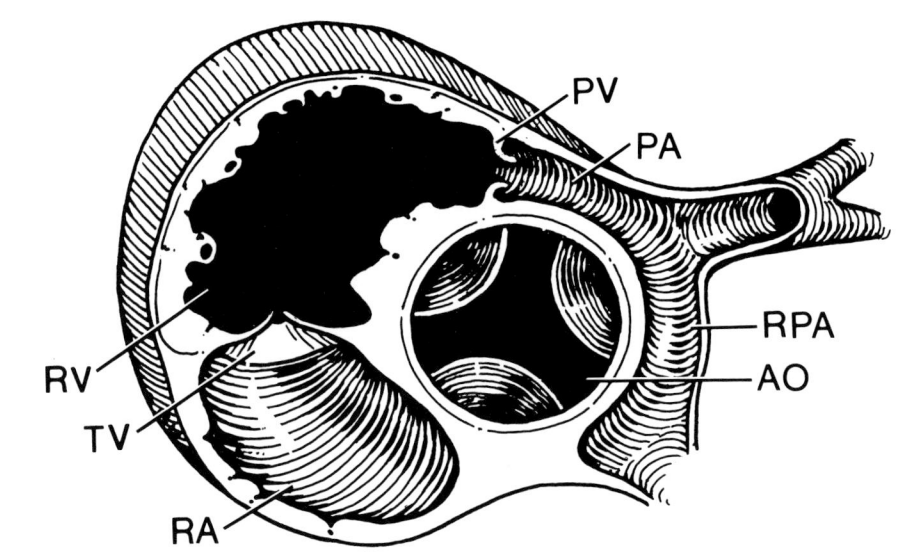

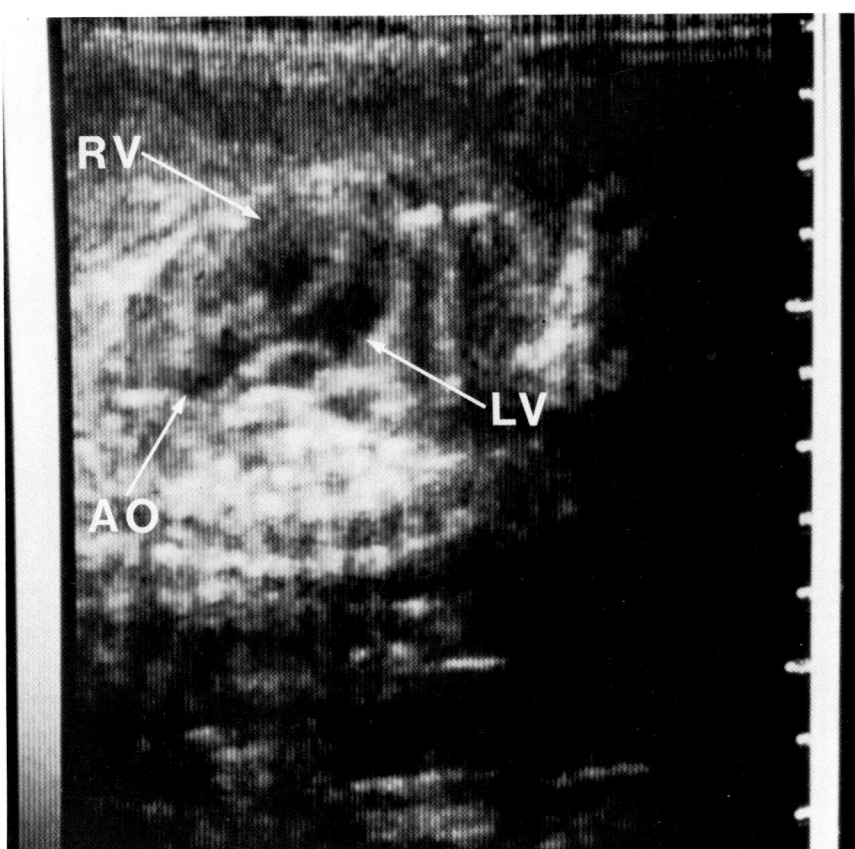

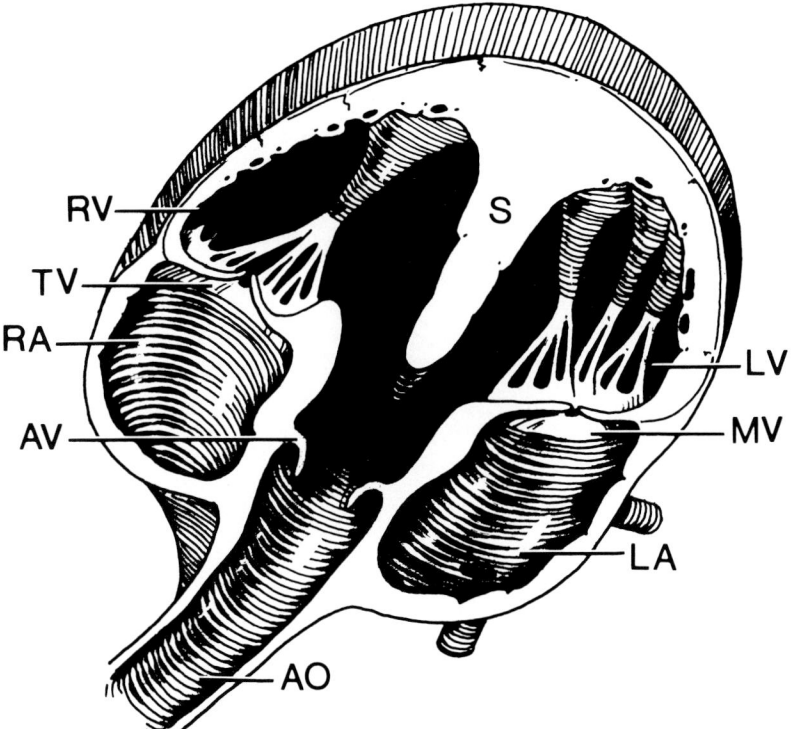

Fig. 4-10c,d. Tetralogy of Fallot. In this five-chamber view of the fetus in Figure 4-10a,b, the ascending aorta (AO) overrides the ventricular septum (S). RV = right ventricle; LV = left ventricle; TV = tricuspid valve; RA = right atrium; AV = aortic valve; MV = mitral valve; LA = left atrium.

(Figure continues on next page.)

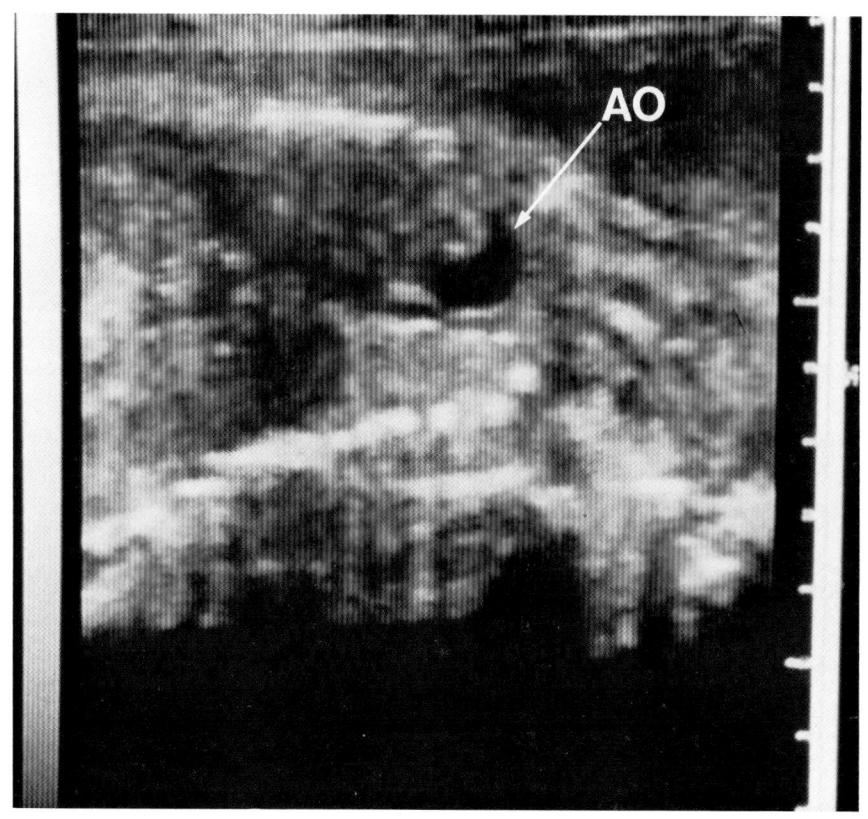

Fig. 4–10e,f. Tetralogy of Fallot. The ascending aorta curves posteriorly in this abbreviated view of the aortic arch (AO) in this fetus presented in Figures 4–10a–d. The ascending portion of the vessel is abnormally dilated but narrows to a more normal diameter as it reaches the posterior aspect of the transverse arch. The fetal head is to the image right. RPA = right pulmonary artery; LA = left atrium; RA = right atrium.

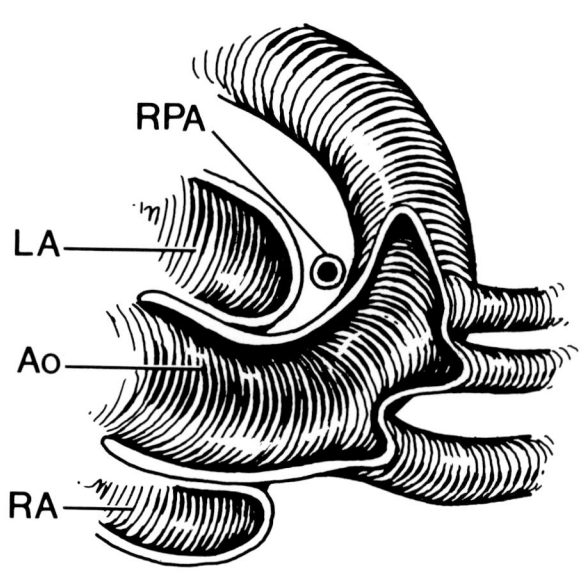

THE ABNORMAL FETAL HEART

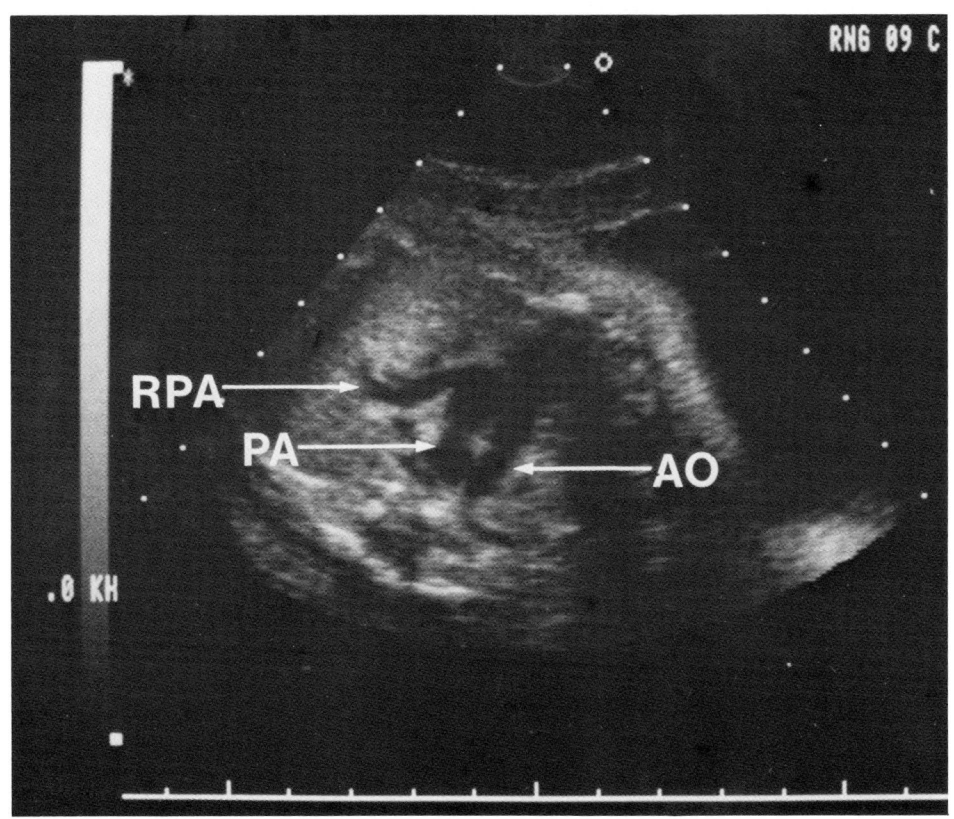

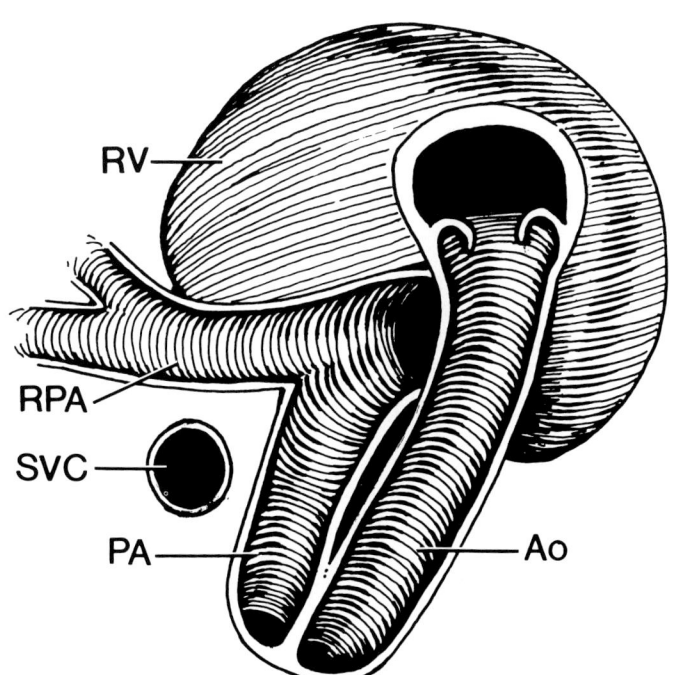

Fig. 4–11a,b. Transposition of the great vessels. The fetus in this image is in a cephalic presentation with the spine at the 7 o'clock position; the scan plane is through the upper thorax. The main pulmonary artery (PA) exits from the left and more posterior ventricle, where it is seen to bifurcate, giving rise to the right pulmonary artery (RPA). The aorta (AO) arises from the anterior ventricle. Other cardiac anomalies in this fetus included tricuspid atresia (Fig. 4–4c), hypoplastic right heart (Fig. 4–2a,b), and ventricular septal defect. This is only one form of transposition of the great vessels. Care must be exercised when examining the aortic arch in apparently normally related great vessels to see that the cerebral vessels arise from the aortic arch. SVC = superior vena cava; RV = right ventricle.

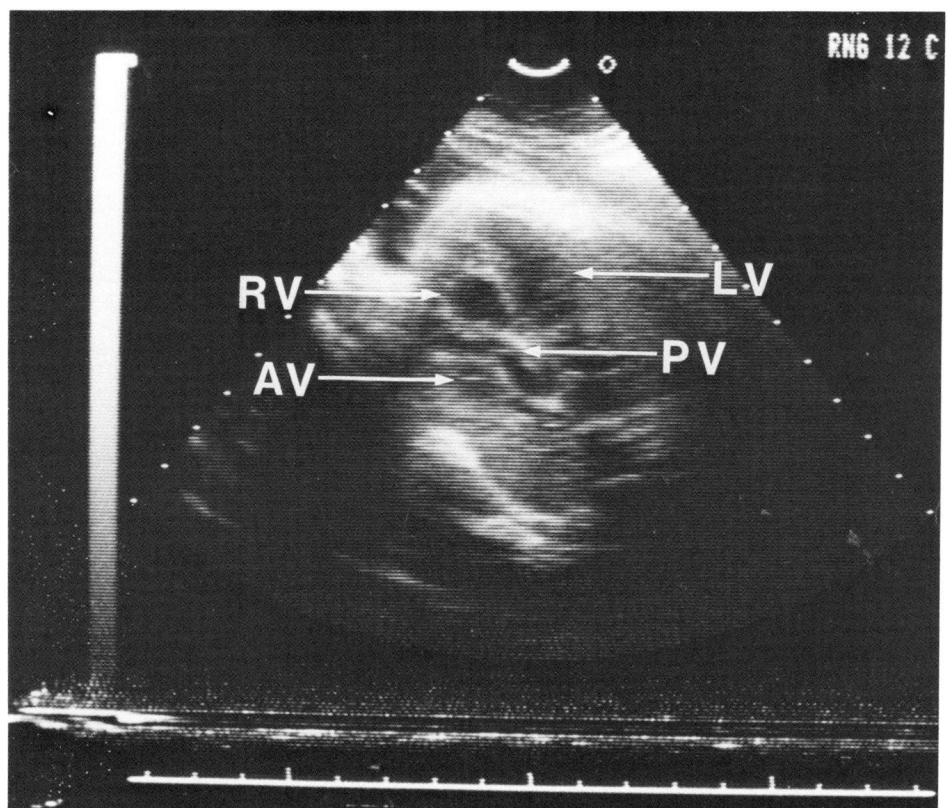

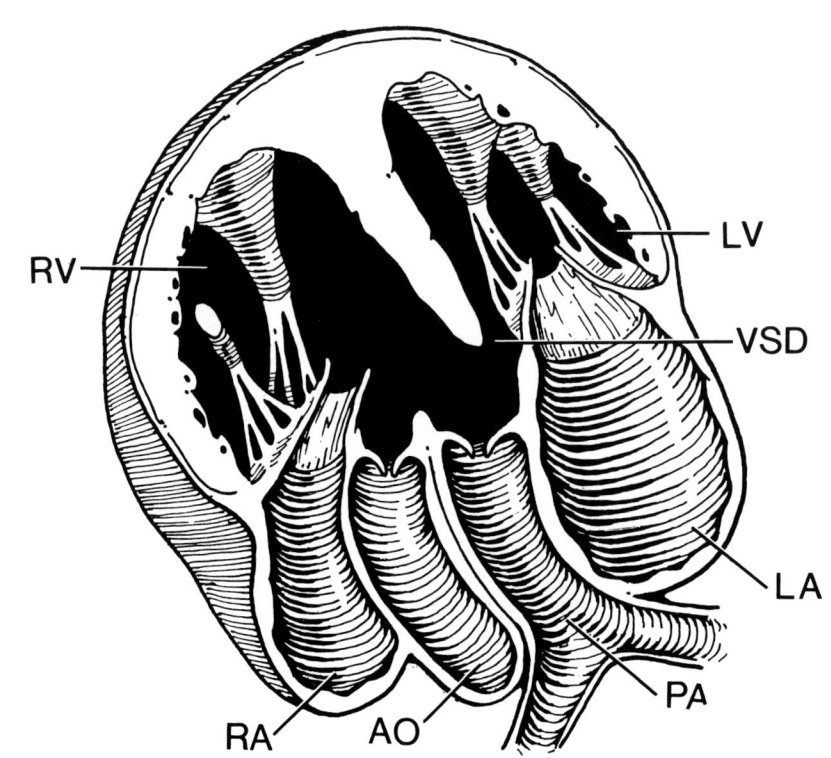

Fig. 4–12a,b. Double-outlet right ventricle. Both great vessels arise from the right side of the heart in this transverse cross-section of the superior aspect of the fetal heart. The fetal spine is at the 4 o'clock position. The aortic valve (AV) is seen to the right of the pulmonary valve (PV). The abnormally positioned ascending aorta in this fetus did not have continuity with the septum. This fetus also had a ventricular and atrial septal defect (Figs. 4–7c and 4–8a). RV = right ventricle; LV = left ventricle; VSD = ventricular septal defect; RA = right atrium; AO = aorta; PA = pulmonary artery; LA = left atrium.

THE ABNORMAL FETAL HEART

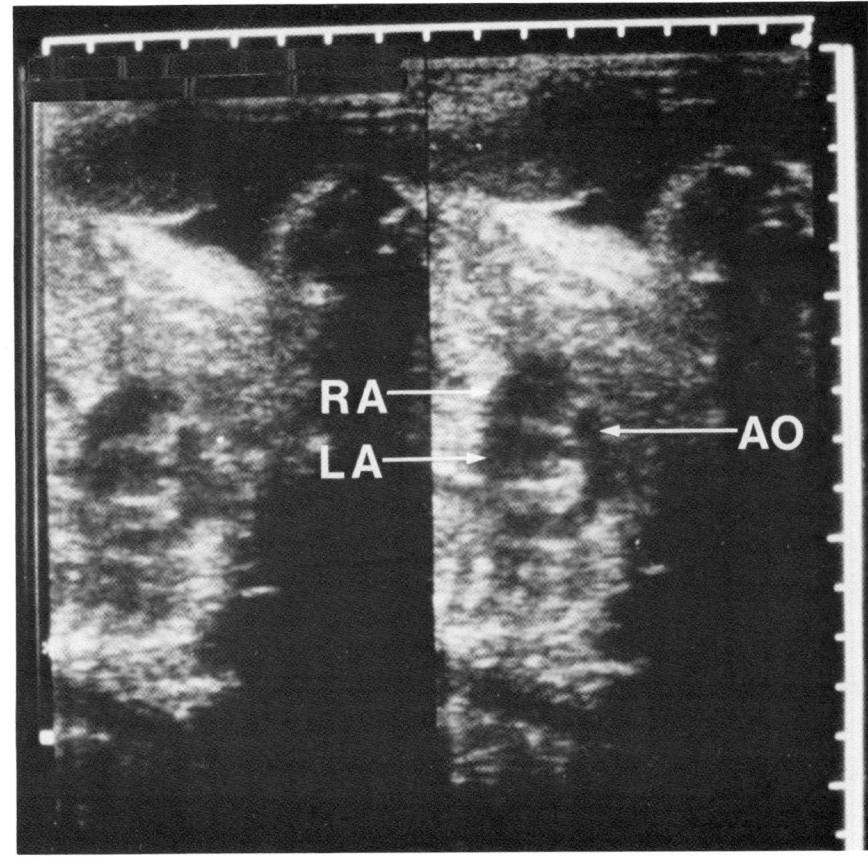

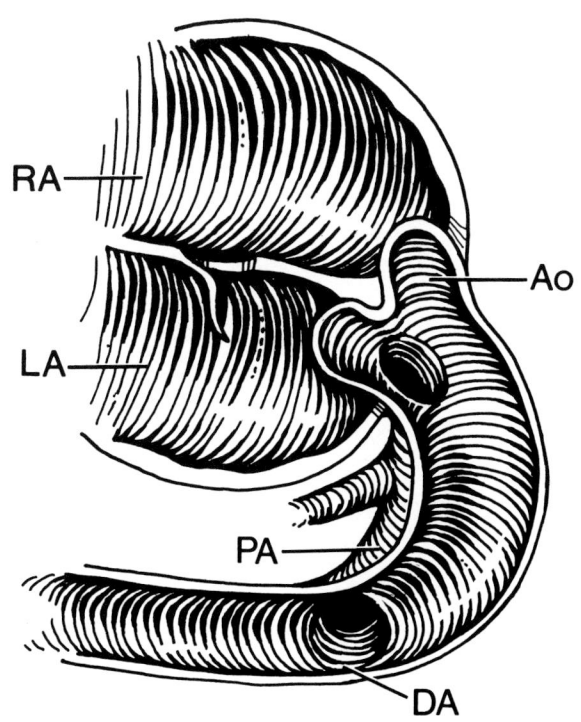

Fig. 4–13a,b. Truncus arteriosus. In this side-by-side long axis image of the aortic arch (AO), the great vessels are anastomosed as they exit the heart. This fetus was also found to have a single ventricle (Fig. 4–3). RA = right atrium; LA = left atrium; PA = pulmonary artery; DA = ductus arteriosus.

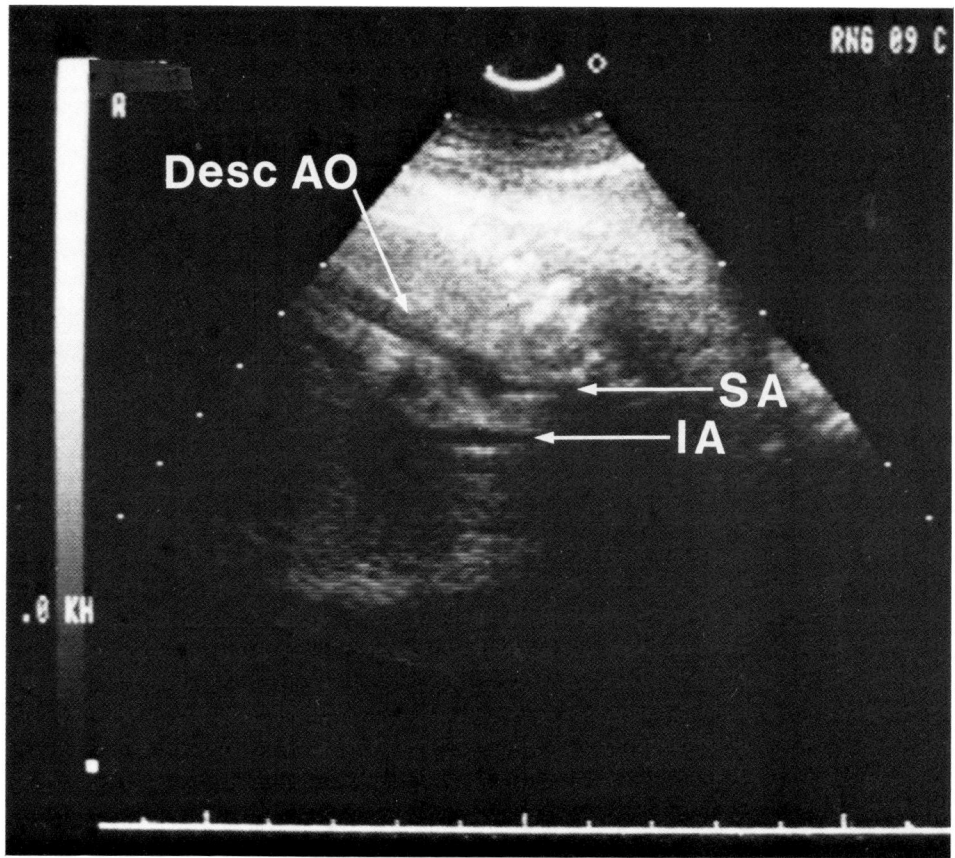

Fig. 4-14a,b. Interrupted aortic arch. The fetal head is to the right of the picture. The innominate artery (IA) can be seen as an extension of the ascending aorta. The left subclavian artery (SA) can be seen as a continuation of the descending aorta. No transverse arch could be seen. A portion of the ductus arteriosus was visualized. At surgery, both carotids arose from the ascending aorta and the two subclavian arteries from the descending aorta. Desc AO = descending aorta; Asc AO = ascending aorta; PA = pulmonary artery.

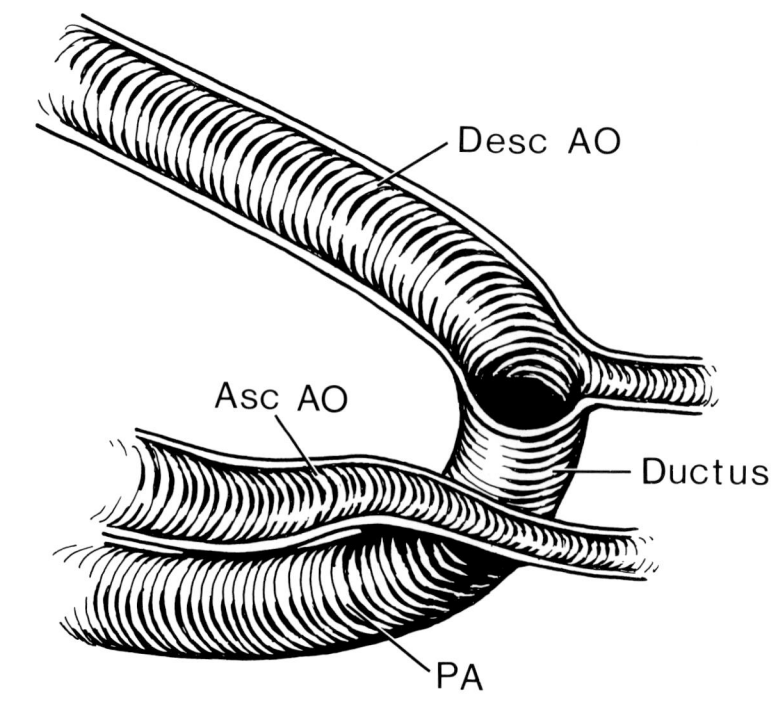

THE ABNORMAL FETAL HEART

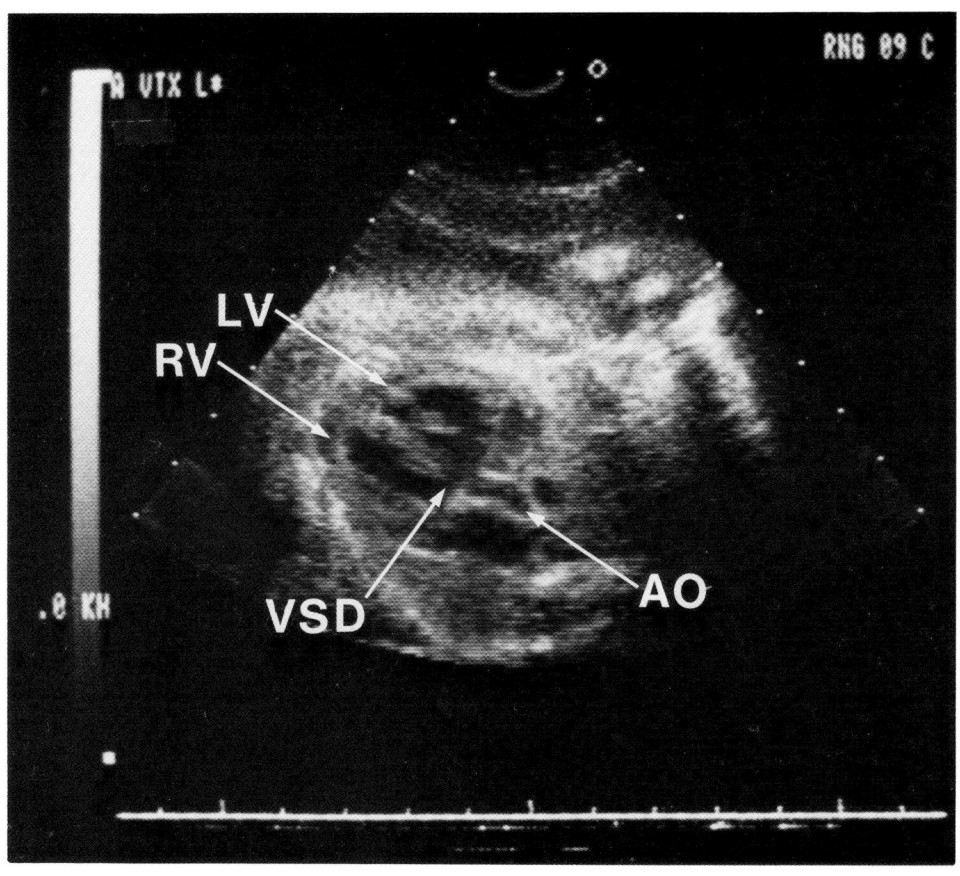

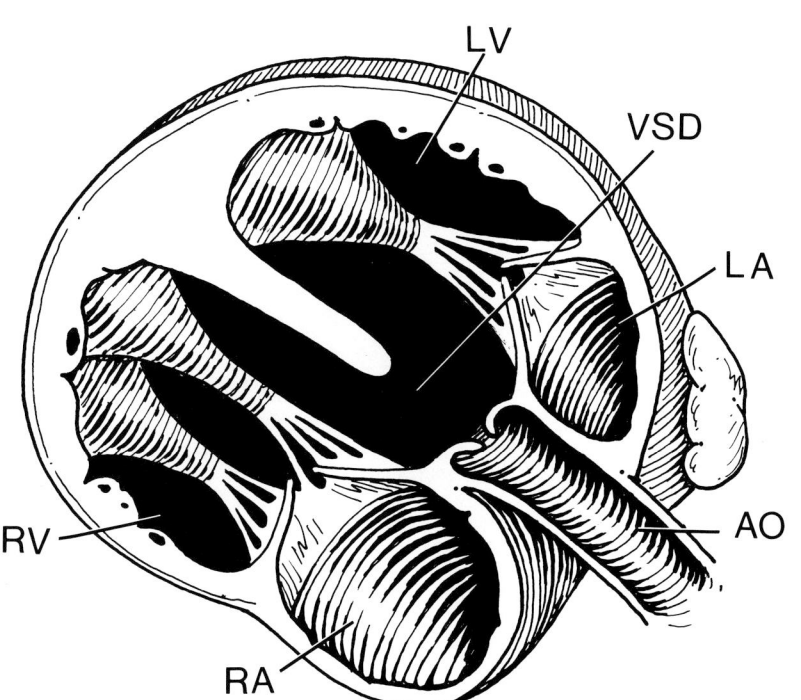

Fig. 4–14c,d. Four-chamber view of the fetus in Figure 4–14a,b with an interrupted aortic arch. The right ventricle is slightly larger than the left ventricle, and a ventricular septal defect (VSD) was also identified. The ascending aorta was abnormally small and subaortic stenosis was present. RV = right ventricle; LV = left ventricle; LA = left atrium; RA = right atrium; AO = aorta.

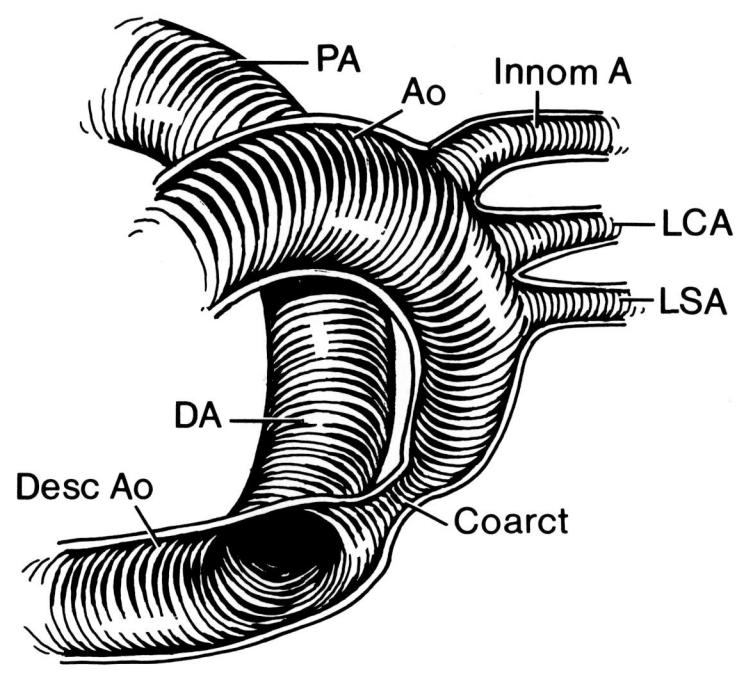

Fig. 4-15. Coarctation of the aorta. In this view the artist depicts a narrowing of the aortic arch between the left subclavian artery (LSA) and the entrance of the ductus arteriosus (DA). Fetal coarctation of the aorta may also be indicated by an enlargement of the right ventricle. PA = pulmonary artery; AO = aortic arch; Innom A = innominate artery; LCA = left carotid artery; Coarct = coarctation; Desc AO = descending aorta.

VEINS

The inferior vena cava may be interrupted, as occurs with left atrial isomerism (Fig. 4-16). A prominent azygous vein may be present also.

The pulmonary veins can be seen entering the left atrium. Anomalous drainage of the pulmonary veins may be apparent in utero; however, since pulmonary blood flow in the fetus is less than in postnatal life, this problem may be more difficult to identify (Fig. 4-17).

THE ABNORMAL FETAL HEART

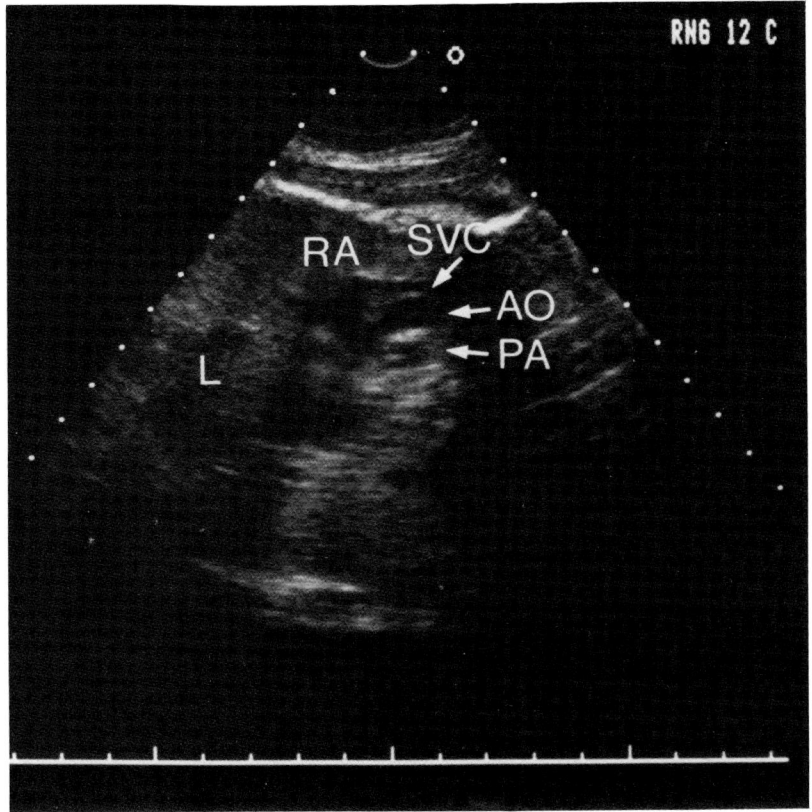

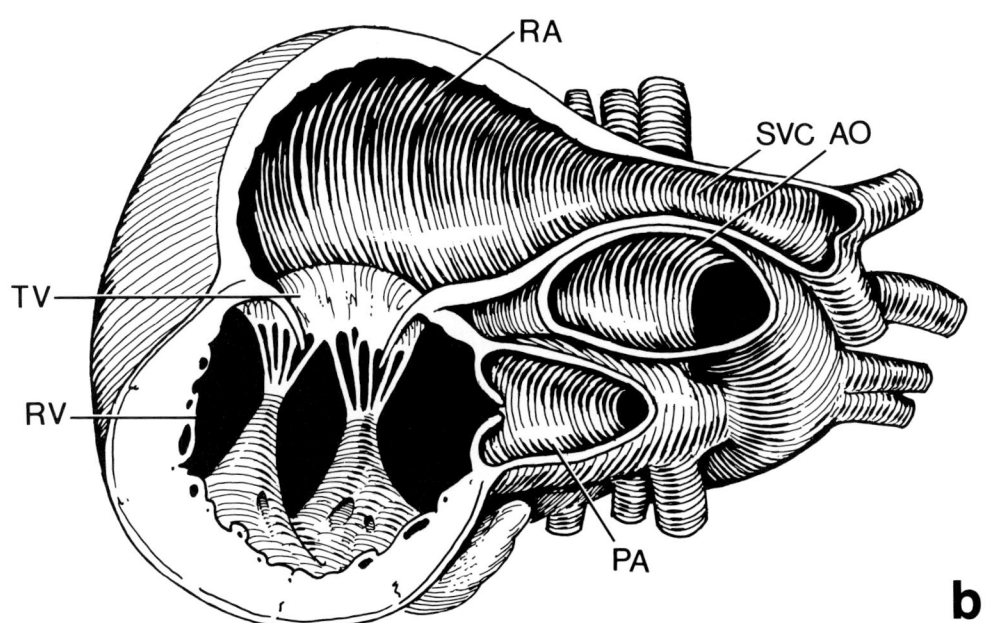

Fig. 4-16a,b. Interrupted inferior vena cava. This is a long axis view of the great vessels from the posterior aspect of the heart in a fetus with an atrioventricular canal defect and left atrial isomerism. The superior vena cava (SVC) enters the right atrium (RA), but there is no connection between the inferior vena cava and the right atrium. The aorta (AO) and pulmonary artery (PA) are positioned normally. (See also Fig. 4-9a,b.) L = liver; TV = tricuspid valve; RV = right ventricle.

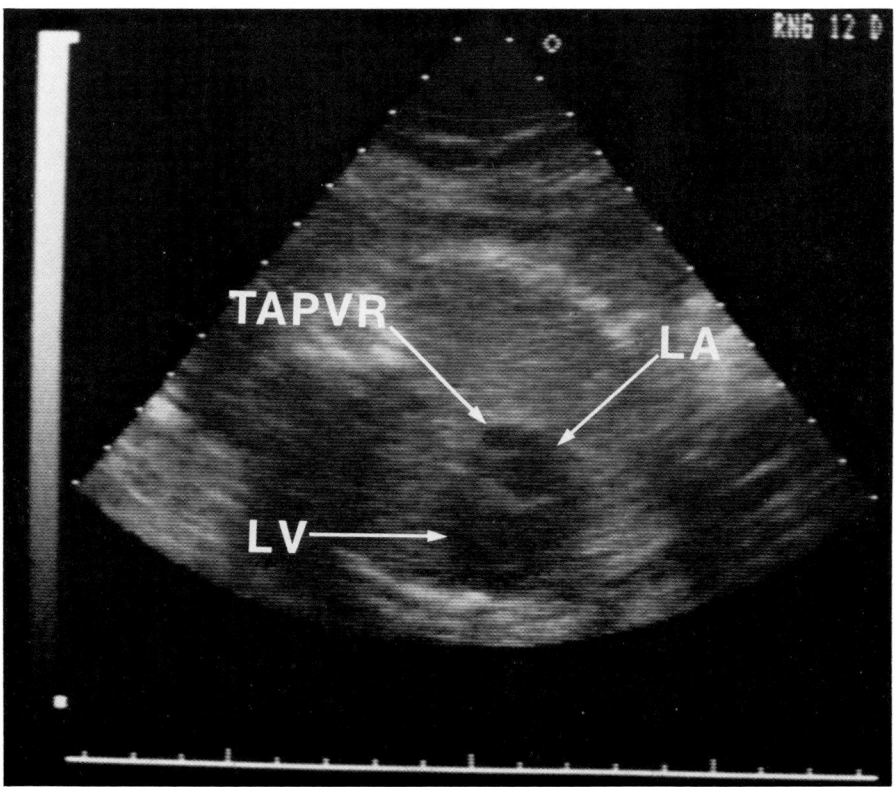

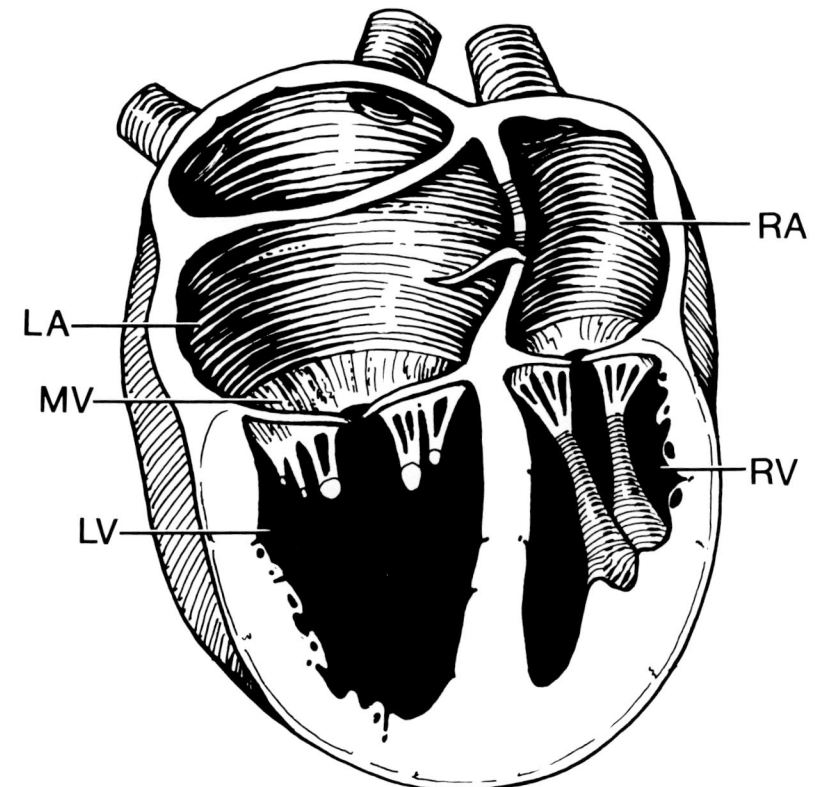

Fig. 4-17a,b. Total anomalous pulmonary venous return (TAPVR). A difficult abnormality to detect; this one was easier in hindsight. The area of entrance of the pulmonary veins into the left atrium (LA) is enclosed by a wall. The pulmonary veins emptied into this conduit and then into the right atrium. The patient was referred for examination for size greater than dates. LV = left ventricle; MV = mitral valve; RA = right atrium; RV = right ventricle.

ABNORMALITIES THAT DEVELOP IN UTERO

Ventricular hypertrophy may develop in utero. This may be a function of prolonged anemia, prolonged increased volume flow (due to a tumor), or it may be idiopathic. Ventricular hypertrophy and pericardial effusions may accompany severe renal anomalies such as infantile polycystic kidneys, multicystic kidneys or renal agenesis (Fig. 4–18). The fetus of a diabetic mother, exposed to hyperglycemia and thus presumably to hyperinsulinemia, may develop an abnormal thickening of the ventricular walls and septum. These features usually resolve postnatally after the environment of the fetus is changed.

Dilatation of the cardiac chambers may occur as part of the presentation of cardiac failure. In the presence of sustained tachyarrhythmias, the right atrium is often dilated, and eventually pericardial and pleural effusions and ascites may develop (Fig. 4–19). Pericardial effusions may accompany any type of congestive heart failure.

Dilatation of the right ventricle followed by dilatation of the left ventricle has been reported in the fetus with severe growth retardation.

Endocardial fibroelastosis is a thickening of the endocardium due to a proliferation of cellular and elastic tissue (Fig. 4–20). It can be associated with obstruction of the great vessels. It is also potentially a familial disorder.

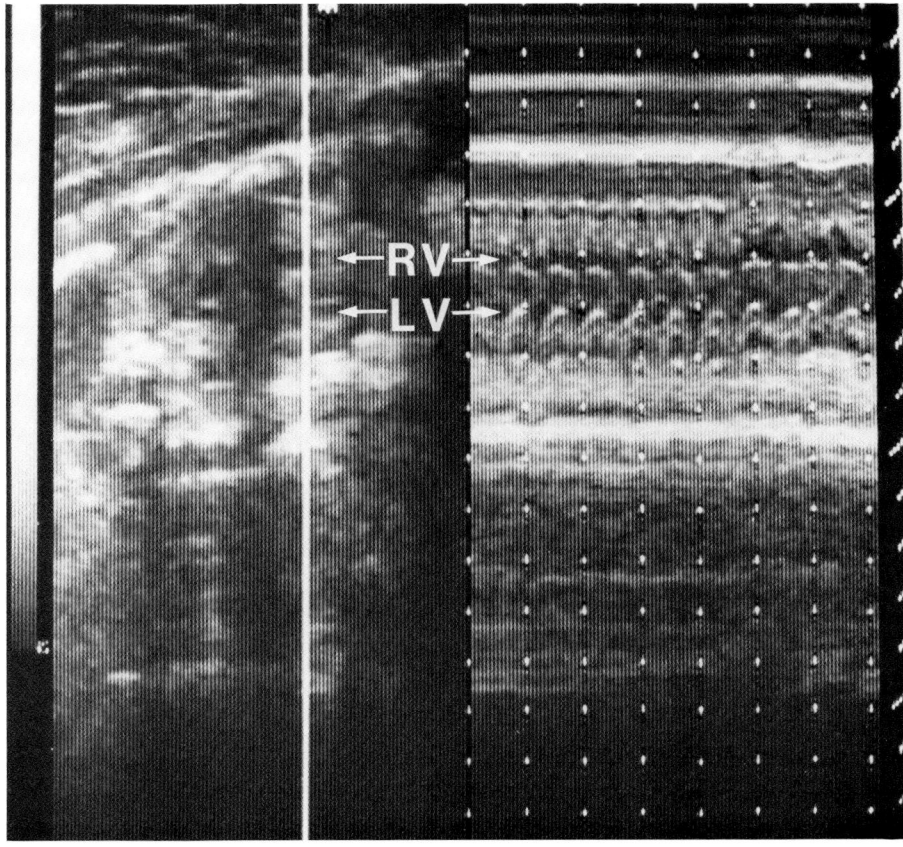

Fig. 4–18a. Ventricular hypertrophy. This is a four-chamber/long axis view of a fetus in a cephalic presentation, with the spine at the 7 o'clock position. The cursor transects the right and left ventricles (RV, LV) below the atrioventricular valves in the two-dimensional image on the left. The right-hand image is the M-mode tracing of the heart at the cursor location. Both ventricular walls and chambers can be measured during systole and diastole. The thickened ventricular septum can also be measured. This patient was referred because multicystic kidneys were found in the fetus during an ultrasound study.

(Figure continues on next page.)

84 FETAL ECHOCARDIOGRAPHY: AN ATLAS

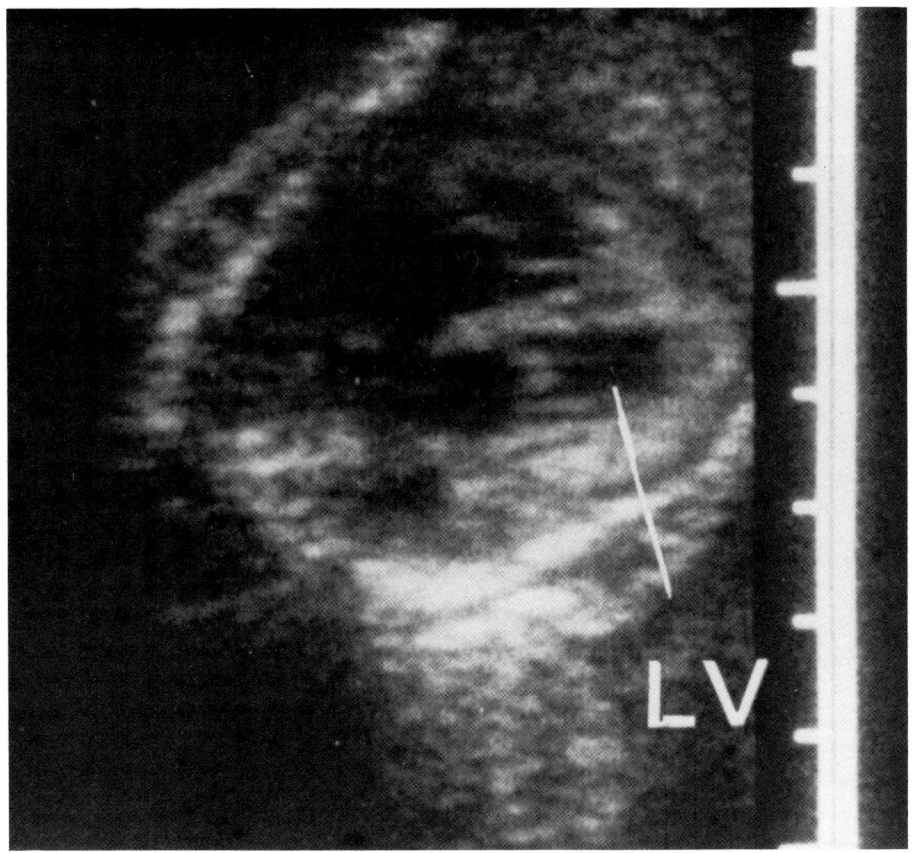

Fig. 4-18b,c. Ventricular hypertrophy. This fetus is in a cephalic presentation, with the spine at the 8 o'clock position. Both ventricular walls are thickened, and the heart occupies most of the chest. The fetus had hypoplastic lungs and severe hemolytic anemia. LV = left ventricle; RV = right ventricle; TV = tricuspid valve; MV = mitral valve; RA = right atrium; FO = foramen ovale; LA = left atrium; S = septum.

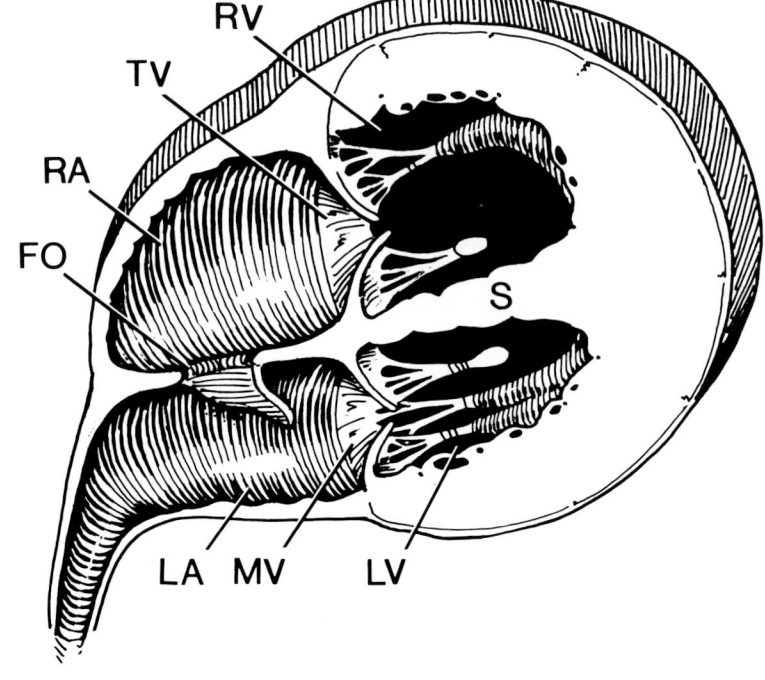

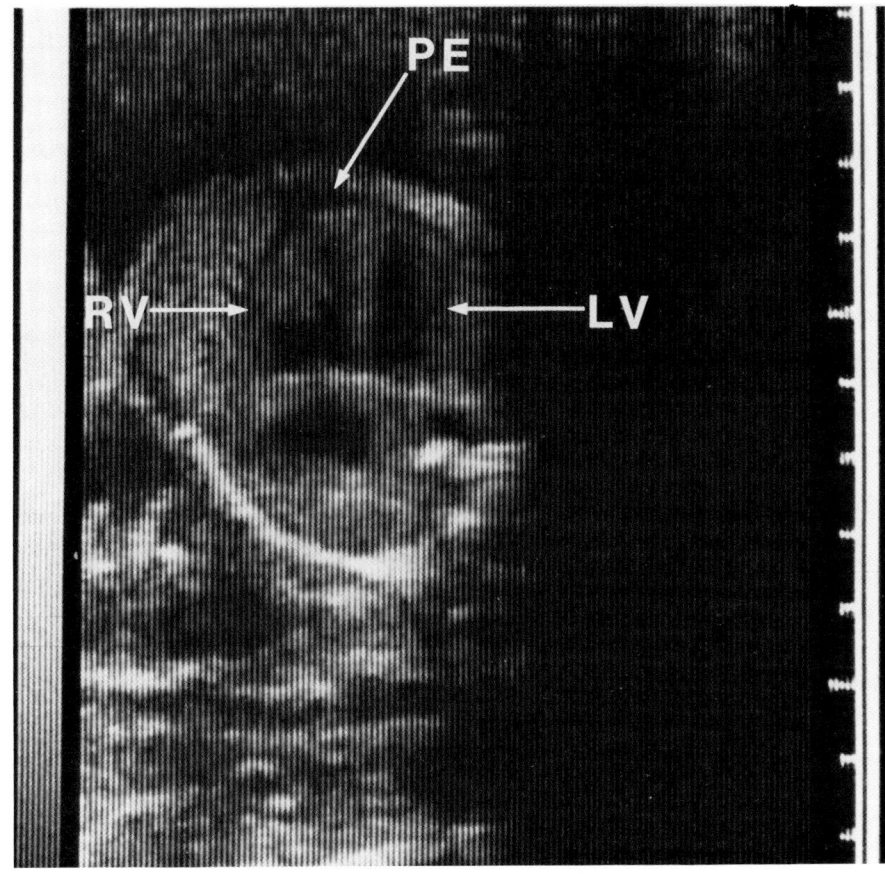

Fig. 4–18d. Ventricular hypertrophy/pericardial effusion. This fetus is in a cephalic presentation with the spine at the 4 o'clock position; the four chambers are seen from the apex. Both right and left ventricles (RV, LV) are enlarged with thickened walls. Right heart enlargement is slightly greater than that of the left, due to cardiac failure. An echo-free zone also present in Figure 4–18b is seen at the apex of the heart and represents a pericardial effusion (PE).

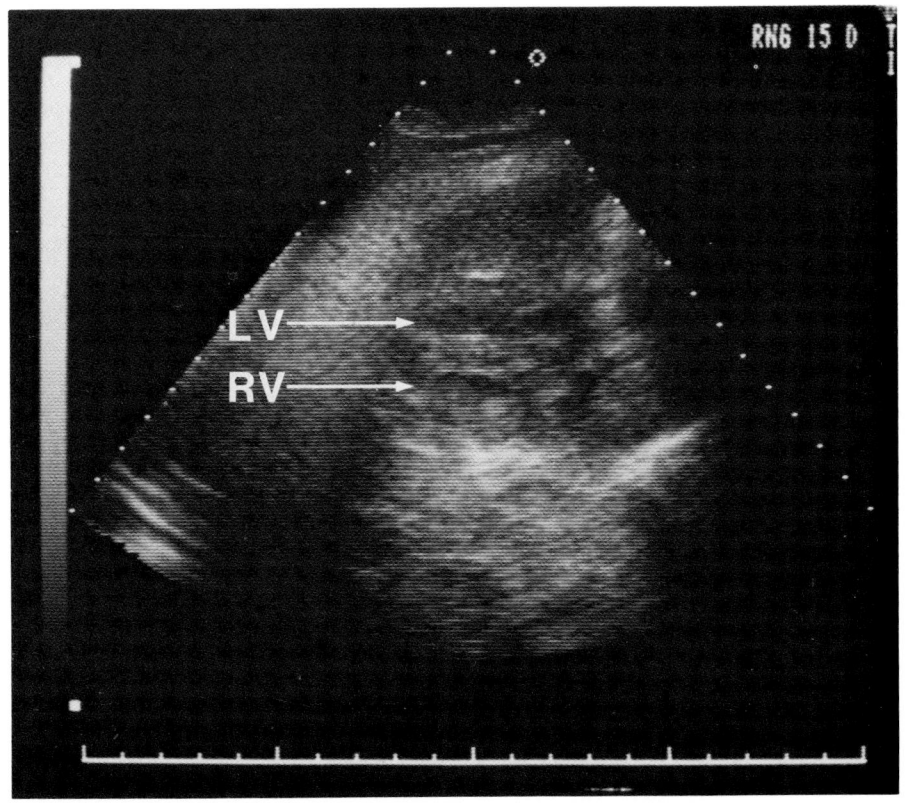

Fig. 4–18e. Septal hypertrophy. In this infant of a class A diabetic mother, the image is of a four-chamber/long axis view, with the spine at the 1 o'clock position. The right and left ventricular (RV, LV) walls are thickened, as is the ventricular septum.

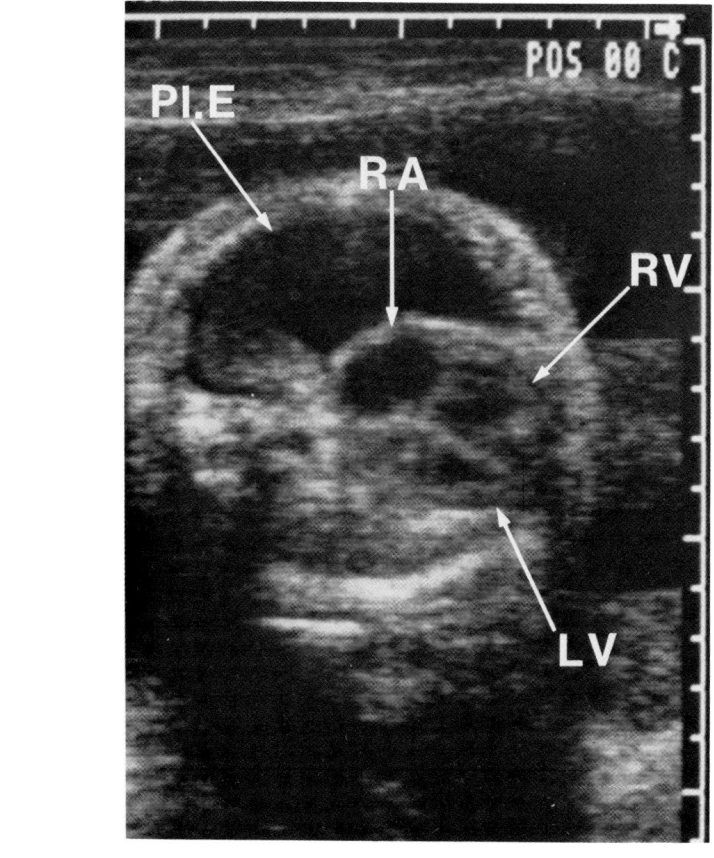

Fig. 4–19a,b. Right heart enlargement. This image is from a patient referred for fetal tachycardia. The fetus is in a cephalic presentation, with the spine at the 9 o'clock position. A large echo-free area to the right of the heart signifies a large pleural effusion (Pl. E). Ascites is also present. The right atrium (RA) and right ventricle (RV) are enlarged due to cardiac failure from the rapid heart rate, which does not allow normal circulation of blood. The mother was treated with digoxin and verapamil and was monitored for several weeks. The fetus converted to normal sinus rhythm, with eventual resolution of ascites and effusions. The patient delivered a normal, healthy infant at term. LV = left ventricle.

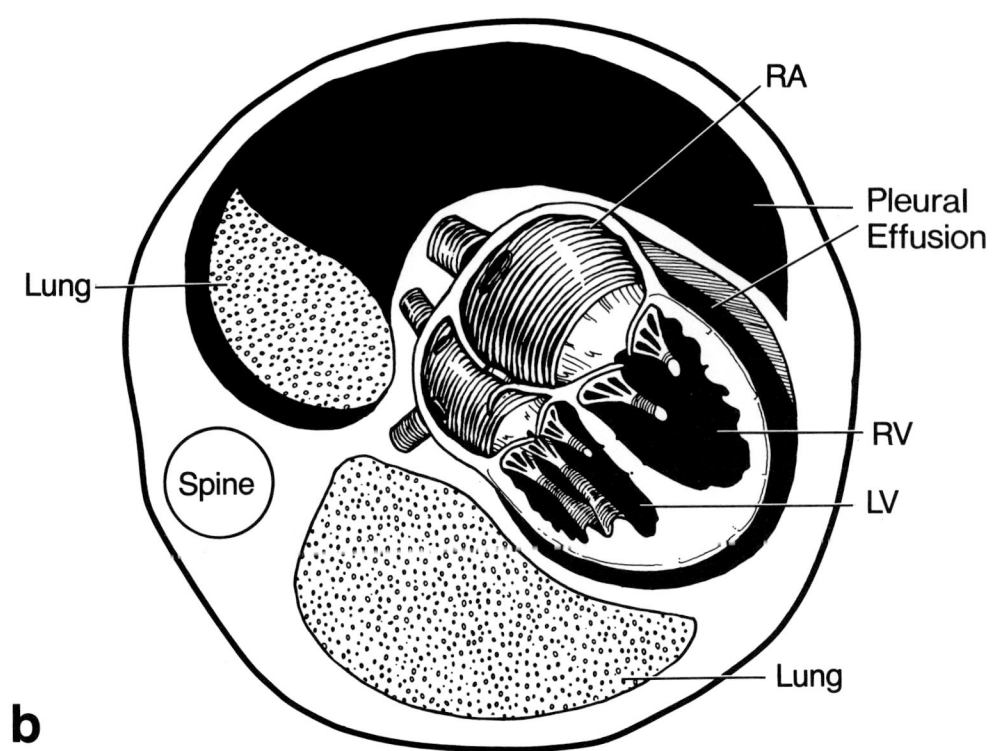

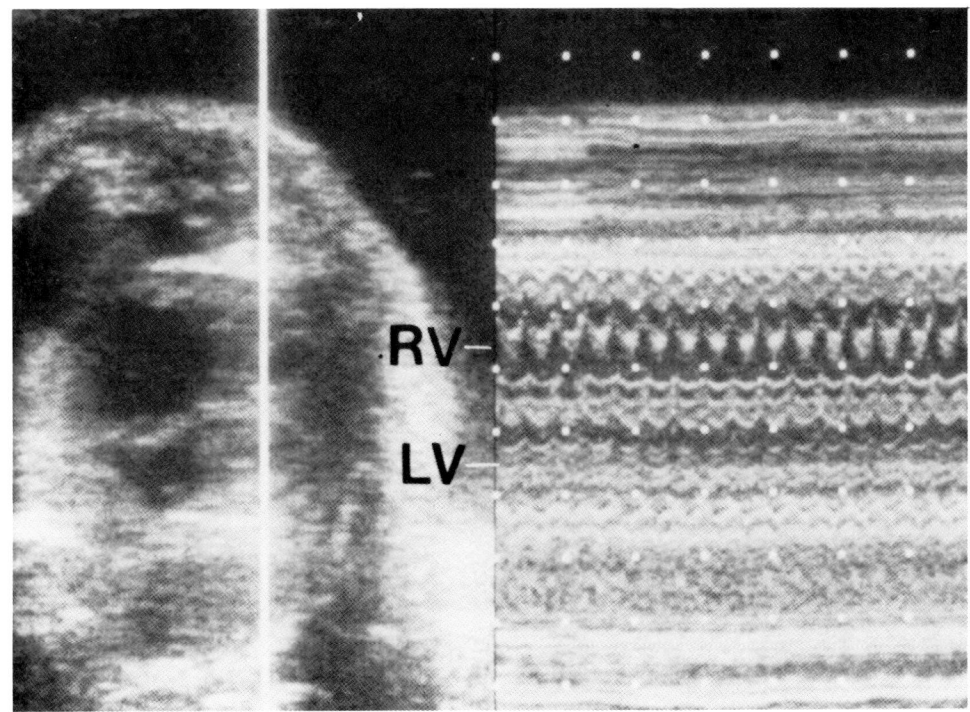

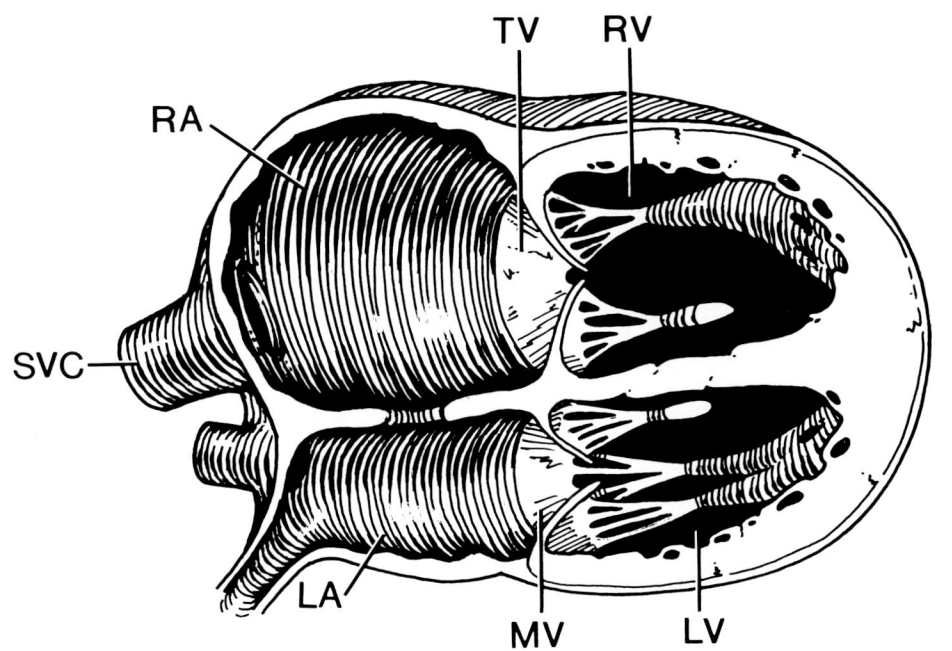

Fig. 4-19c,d. Cardiac failure with supraventricular tachycardia. This fetus is in a cephalic presentation with the spine at the 8 o'clock position. An M-mode tracing from the region designated by the cursor is seen to the right of the image (heart rate 300 bpm). A small pericardial effusion is visible inferior to the left ventricle (LV). This fetus converted to normal sinus rhythm at delivery by cesarean and did well on digoxin after birth. RV = right ventricle; TV = tricuspid valve; MV = mitral valve; RA = right atrium; LA = left atrium; SVC = superior vena cava.

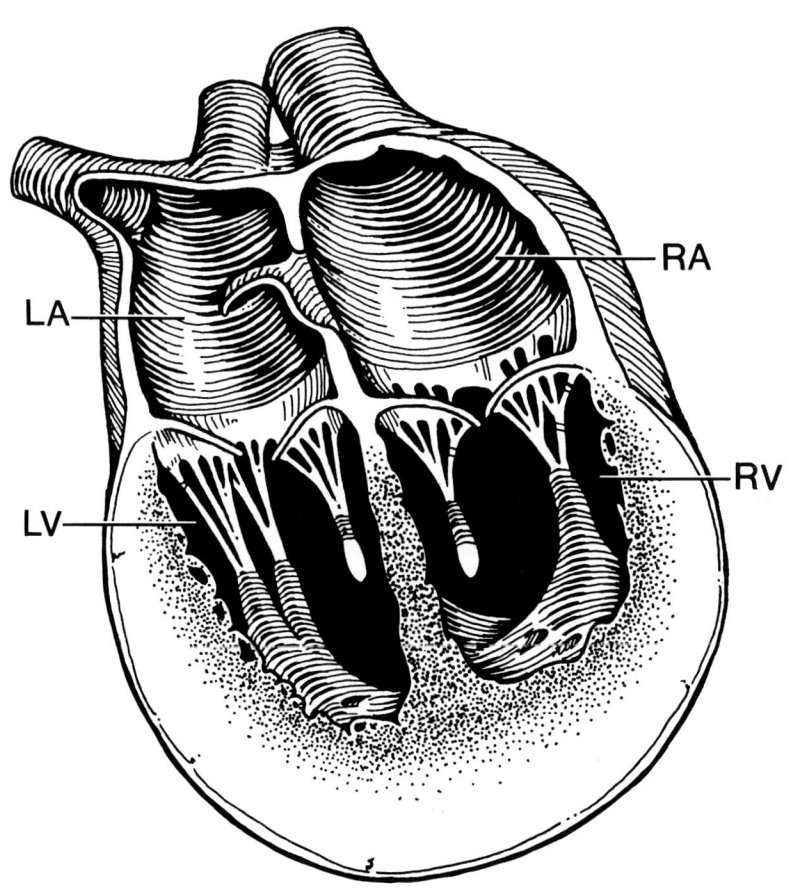

Fig. 4-20. Endocardial fibroelastosis. This occurs in the presence of a proliferation of cellular and elastic tissue. An ultrasound image would show bright echogenic areas within the ventricular walls. RA = right atrium; LA = left atrium; RV = right ventricle; LV = left ventricle.

OTHER TYPES OF CARDIAC ABNORMALITIES

Abnormalities of cardiac rhythm that result in unusual blood flow patterns may temporarily distort the appearance of the fetal heart (Fig. 4-21).

Tumors may occur in the fetal heart (Fig. 4-22). These include rhabdomyomas, which may occur with tuberous sclerosis, and teratomas. Abnormalities of blood flow and arrhythmias may acompany these tumors.

The fetal heart may not be located normally within the fetal chest. Situs inversus, with various accompanying cardiac and visceral manifestations, may be present (Fig. 4-23). The fetal heart may be shifted by the presence of a diaphragmatic hernia (Fig. 4-24), congenital lobar emphysema (Fig. 4-25), or cystic adenomatoid malformation of the lung.

The heart may be located externally to the chest (ectopia cordis, Fig. 4-26).

Twins are another potentially complicating factor. A greater incidence of malformations is present in twins. Twin-twin transfusion may occur (Fig. 4-27). This can be investigated by measuring the fetal sizes and by identifying the intervening membrane. Doppler blood flows may give further indication of fetal abnormalities. Twins may also be conjoined (Fig. 4-28).

Umbilical cord examination should also be performed. Identification of a two-vessel cord should prompt an even more thorough examination for anomalies and follow-up studies for the development of intrauterine growth retardation (Fig. 4-29).

SUMMARY

The approach to the abnormal fetal heart may be quite varied. There may be suspicion of an abnormality at the time of examination, such as in the presence of a known chromosome abnormality, or a fetus with hydrops or other identified abnormalities on ultrasound. The examination may be one done for fetal measurement, and an abnormality may be discovered as part of a screening examination. The mother may fall into a high-risk category (see Introduction).

It is important to have sufficient time and expertise to methodically investigate all the features of the fetus and of the heart. The term "segmental" examination is used frequently and should be emphasized. With this approach, each segment of the fetal heart is thoroughly examined so that no abnormalities are overlooked.

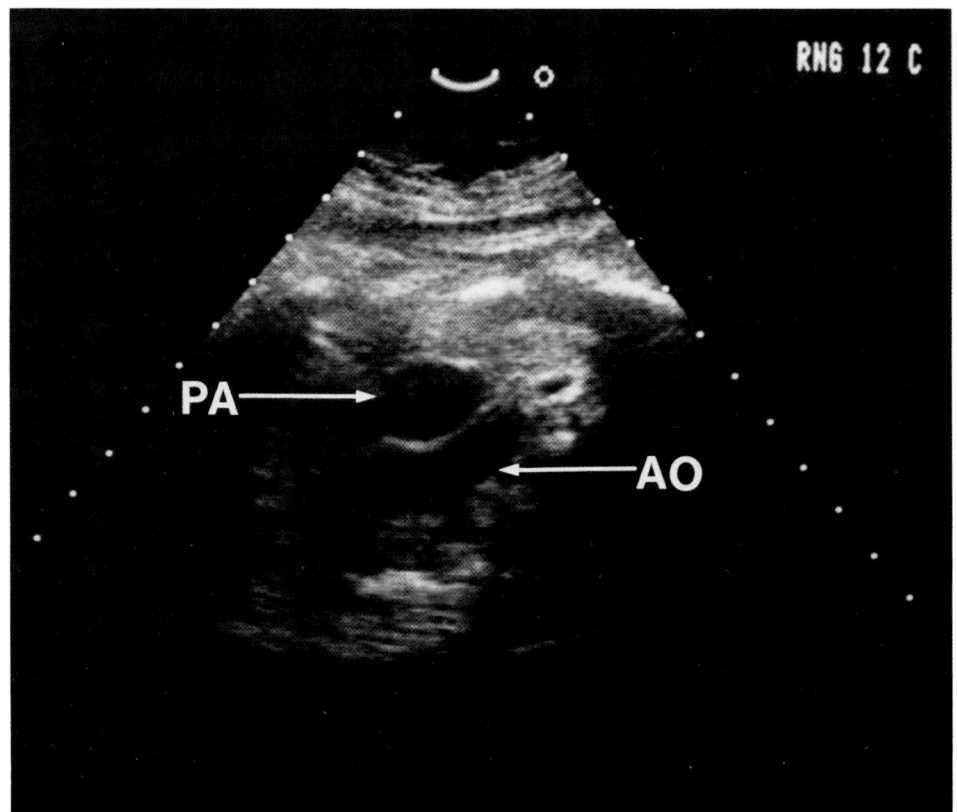

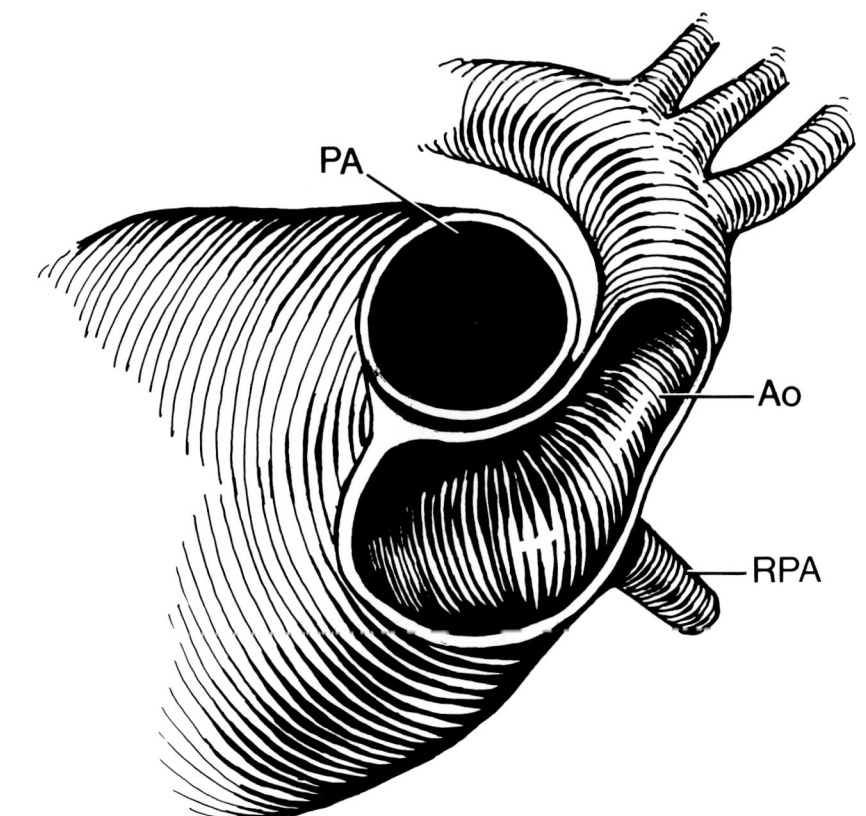

Fig. 4-21a,b. Complete heart block. The pulmonary artery (PA) of a fetus with complete heart block (mother was anti-Ro antibody positive) is shown in cross section, with a lateral view of the transverse aortic arch (AO) crossing on the fetal right. Both vessels were dilated during systole. RPA = right pulmonary artery.

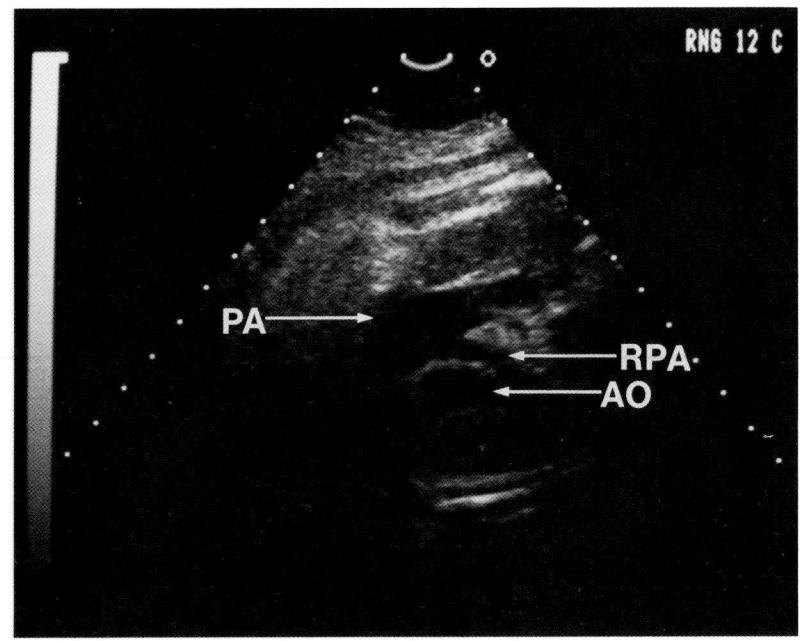

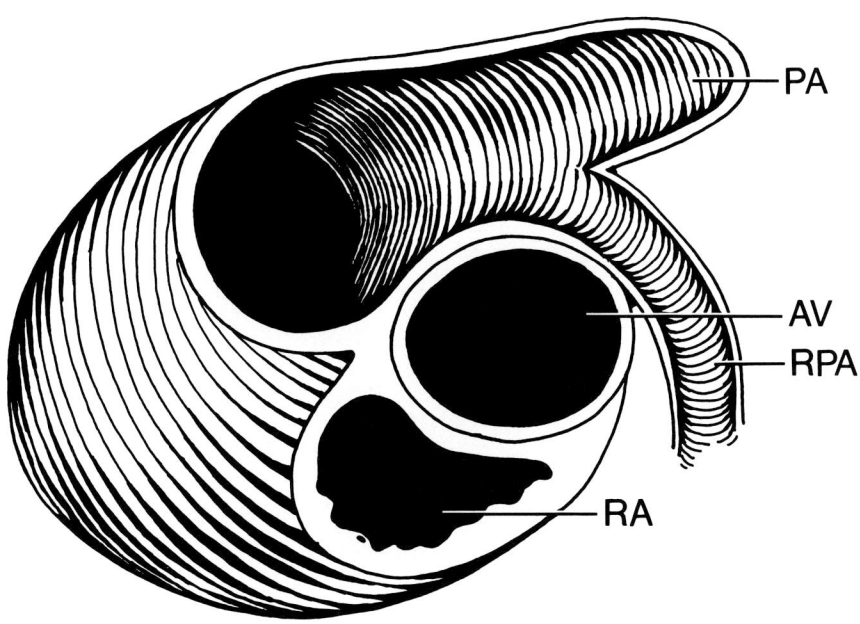

Fig. 4-21c,d. Complete heart block. This short axis view of the great vessels is at 90 degrees to the view seen in Figure 4-21a,b. This again demonstrates dilatation of the great vessels during heart block. PA = pulmonary artery; RPA = right pulmonary artery; AO = aorta; AV = aortic valve; RA = right atrium.

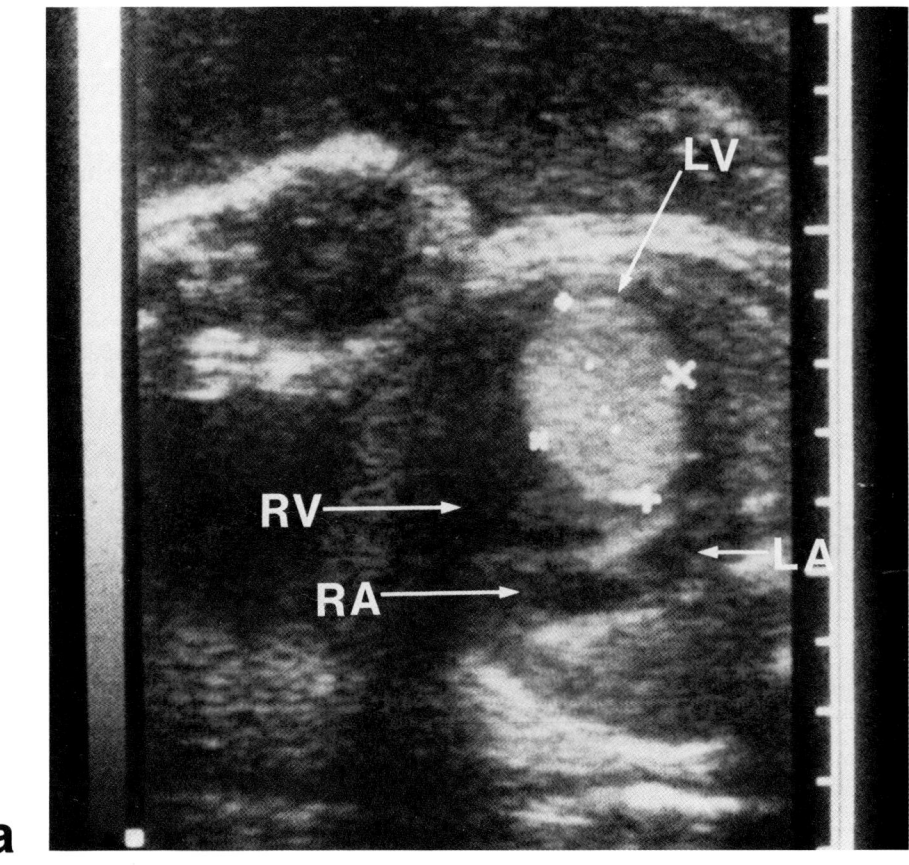

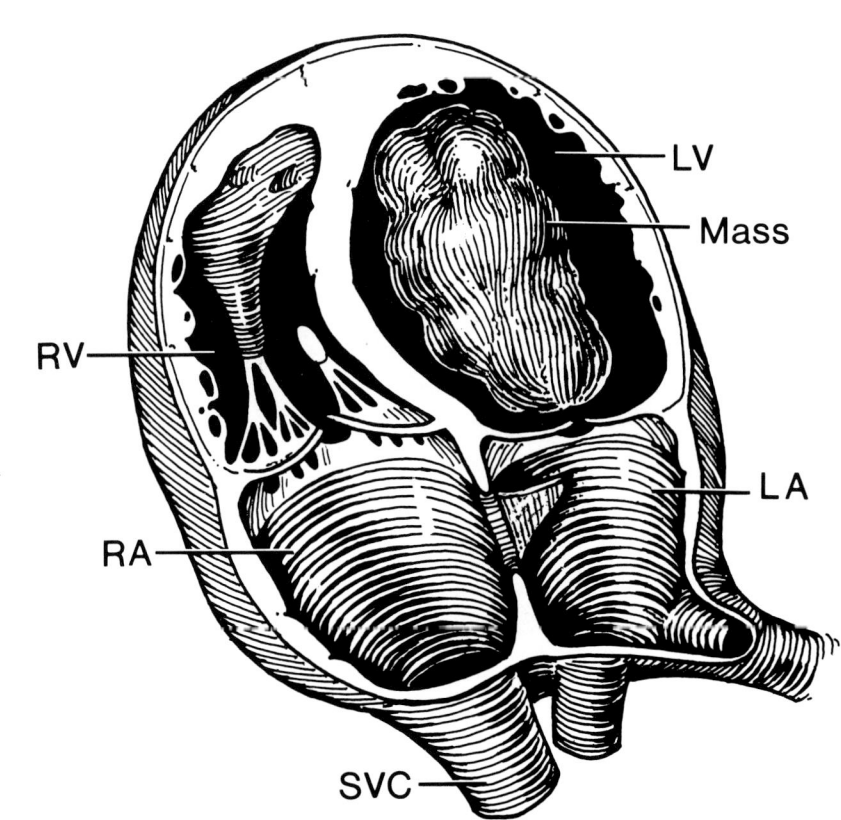

Fig. 4–22a,b. Cardiac tumor. This patient was referred because of the presence of a fetal cardiac mass. In this apical four-chamber view of the fetus in a cephalic presentation, a large, echo-dense mass fills the left ventricle (LV) deforming the right ventricle (RV). Flow into and out of both chambers was demonstrated utilizing Doppler ultrasound studies. The infant was delivered at term and found to have a rhabdomyoma at surgery. RA = right atrium; LA = left atrium; SVC = superior vena cava.

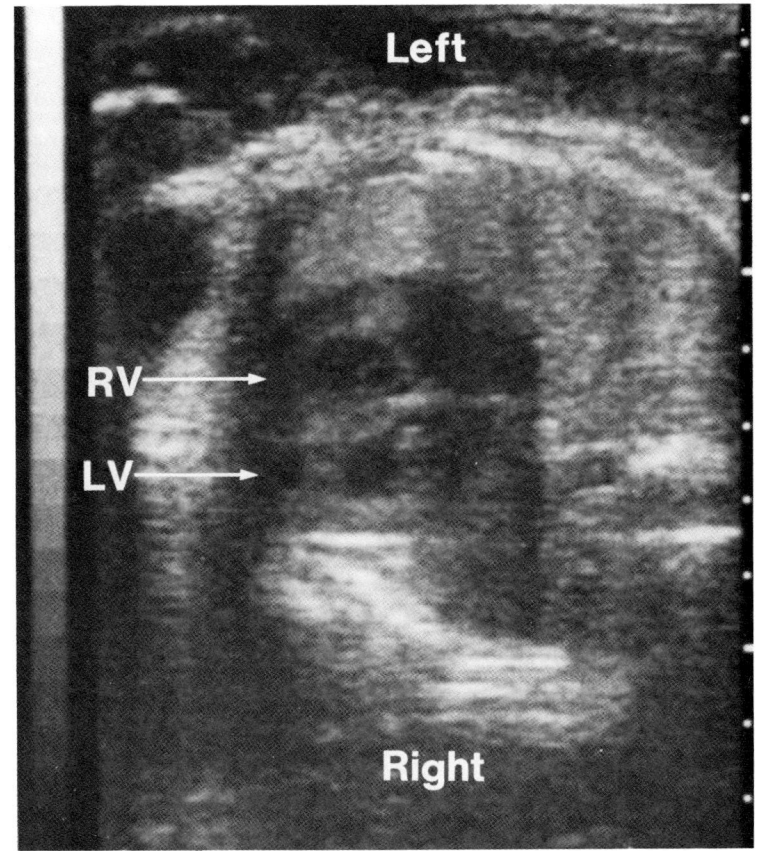

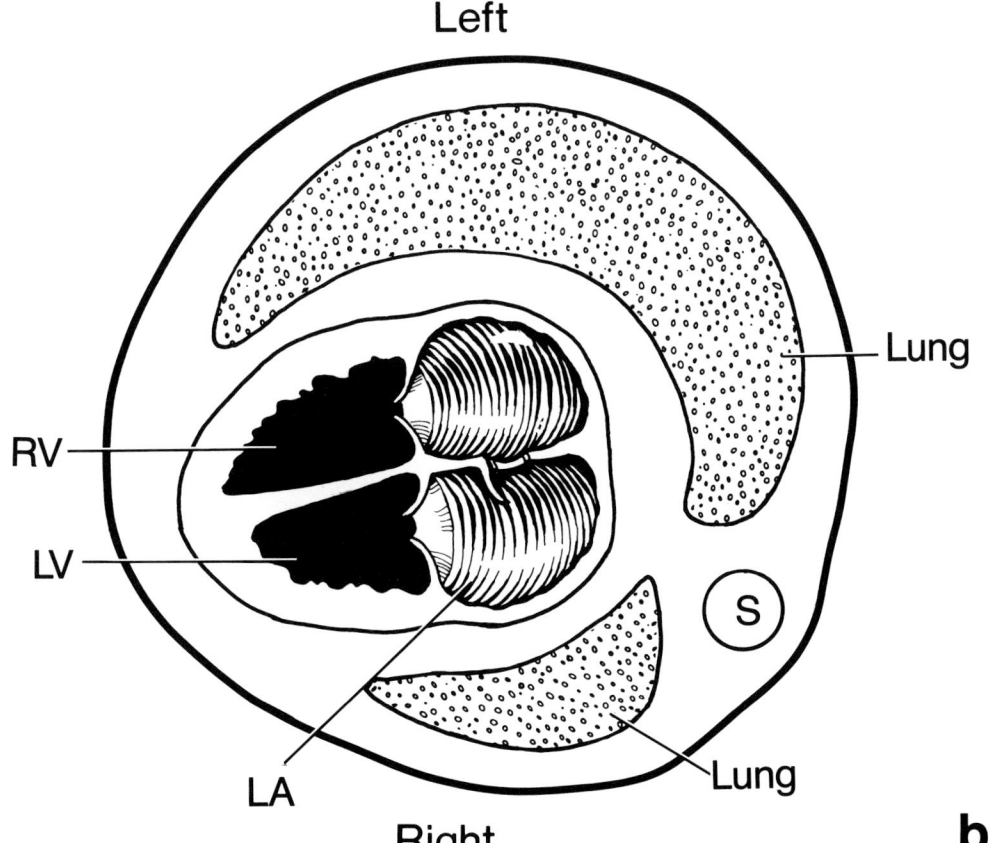

Fig. 4-23a,b. Situs inversus. This patient demonstrates the importance of determining the right and left side of the fetus prior to fixing positions of abdominal and thoracic organs. The fetus is in a cephalic presentation with the spine at the 4 o'clock position. This is a case of complete situs inversus in which all abdominal and thoracic structures were reversed, without evidence of any other abnormality. The patient had been referred for routine examination to document gestational age. RV = right ventricle; LV = left ventricle; LA = left atrium; S = spine.

(Figure continues on next page.)

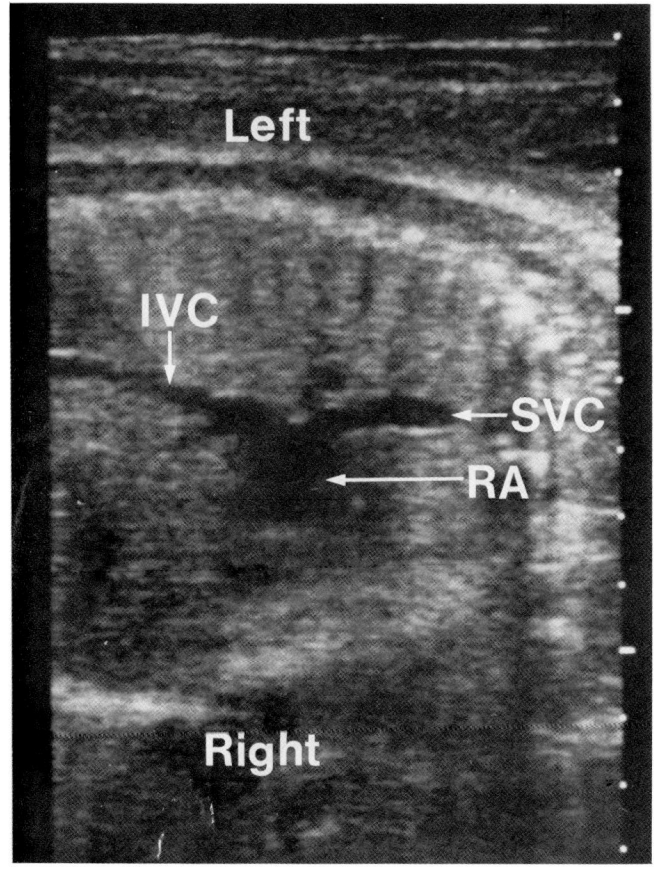

Fig. 4-23c. Situs inversus. In this sagittal view of the fetus shown in Figure 4-23a,b, the ultrasound beam transects the fetus from the left posterior aspect; normally, it should cross through the left atrium and left ventricle. Instead, the beam transects the right heart structures of inferior and superior venae cavae (IVC, SVC) as they enter the right atrium (RA).

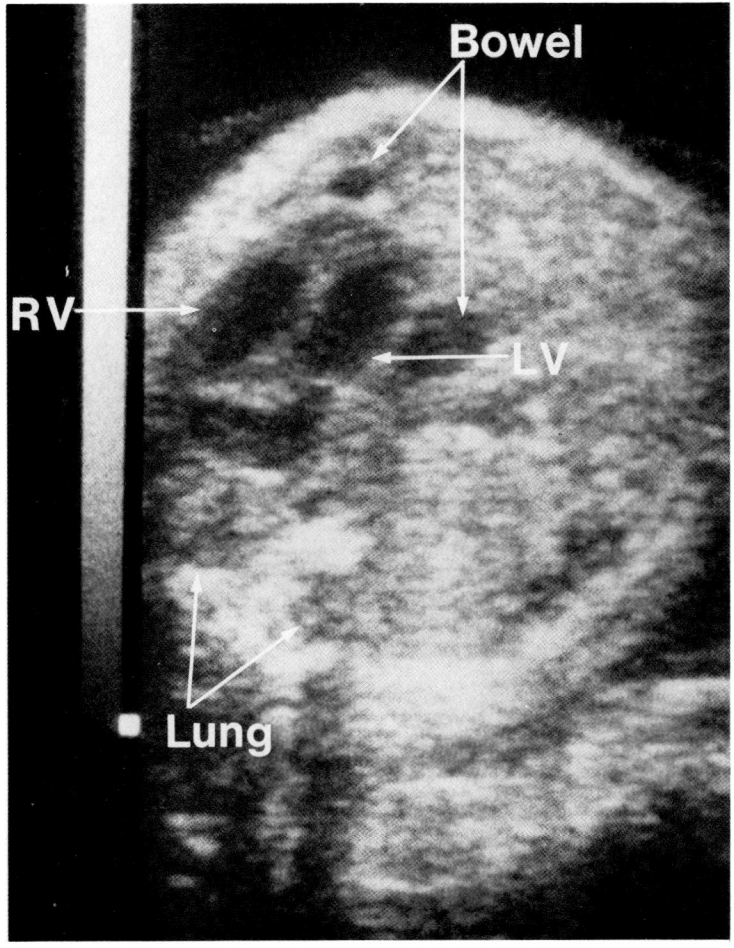

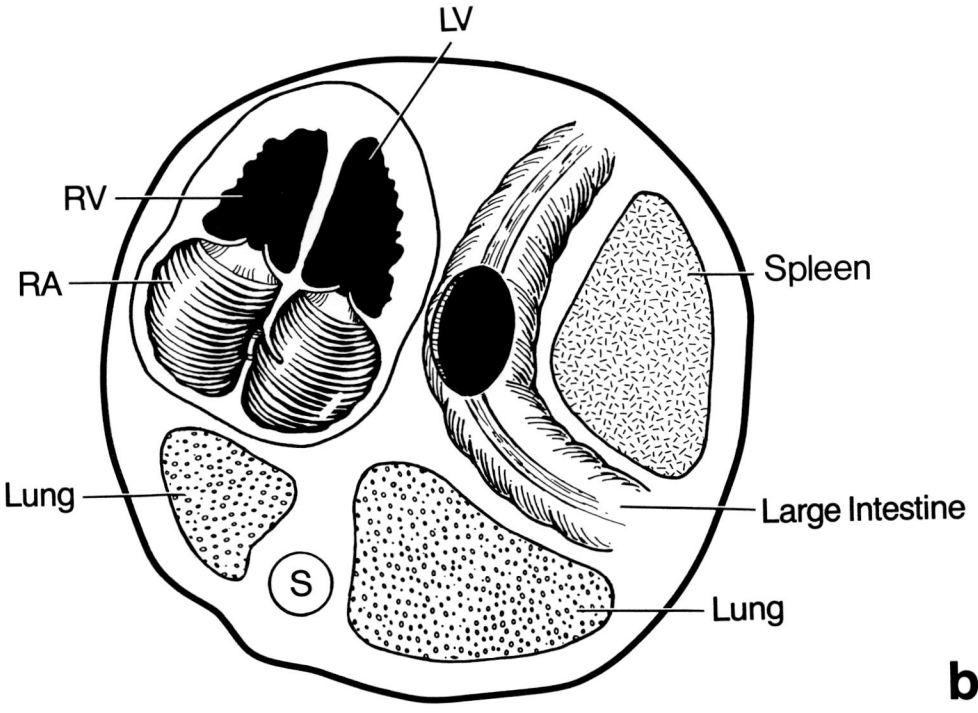

Fig. 4-24a,b. Malposition. Another instance of malposition of the fetal heart is shown in this fetus with congenital diaphragmatic hernia referred for routine dating. The fetus is in a cephalic presentation, with the spine at the 7 o'clock position. Herniation of the stomach, large and small bowel, spleen, and part of the liver through a left posterolateral defect have shifted the heart to the far right chest wall. Pulmonary hypoplasia resulted, from which the infant died shortly after birth. An atrial septal defect also was present (see Fig. 4-8b). RV = right ventricle; LV = left ventricle; RA = right atrium; S = spine.

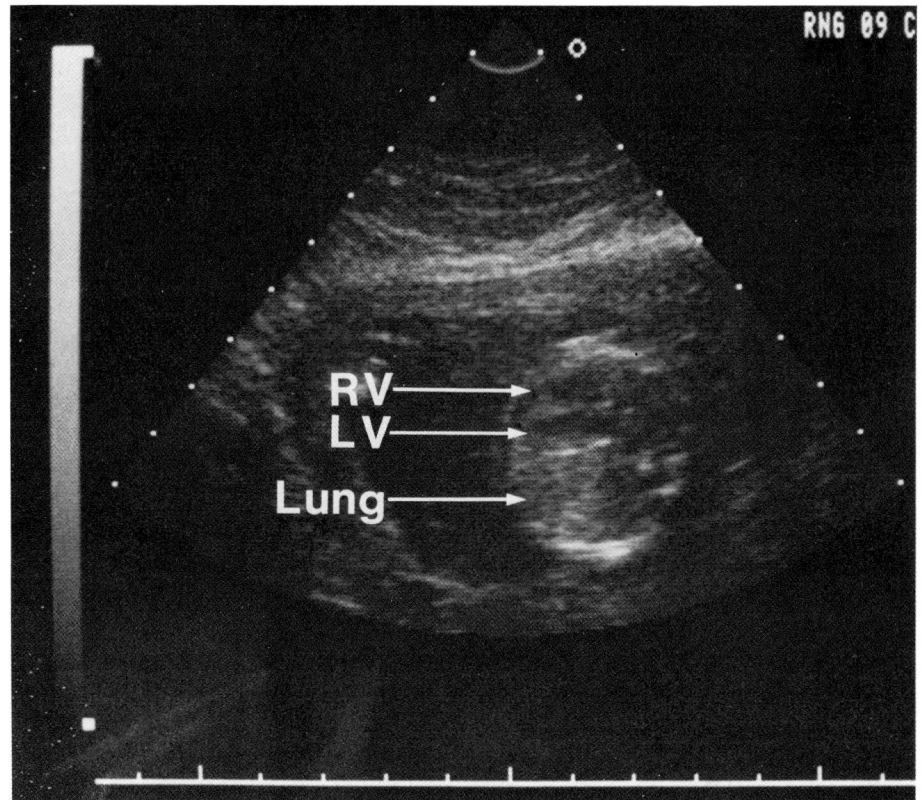

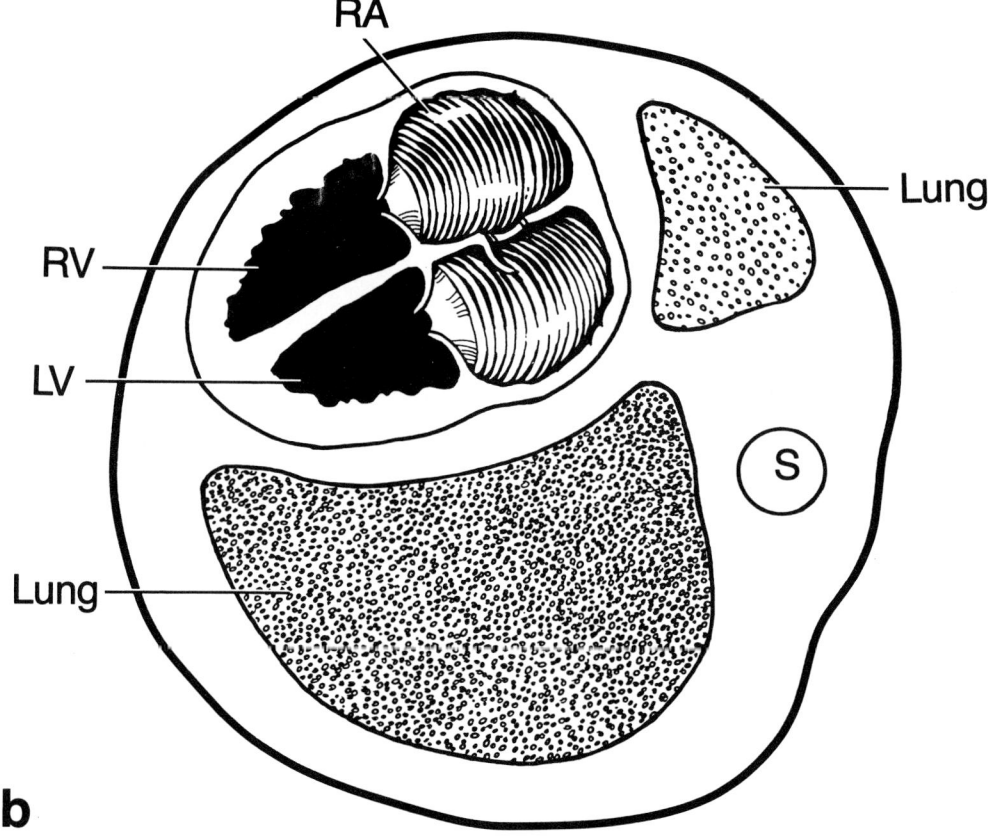

Fig. 4–25a,b. Malposition. Lung pathology such as cystic adenomatoid malformation, lung tumors, and, as in this fetus, congenital lobar emphysema, can also cause a shift in heart position. The left lung in this fetus was slightly more echo dense than normal, and a small cystic structure was seen posteriorly. The mother's previous infant died of hypoplastic left heart syndrome. This baby did well throughout fetal and neonatal life. RV = right ventricle; LV = left ventricle; RA = right atrium; S = spine.

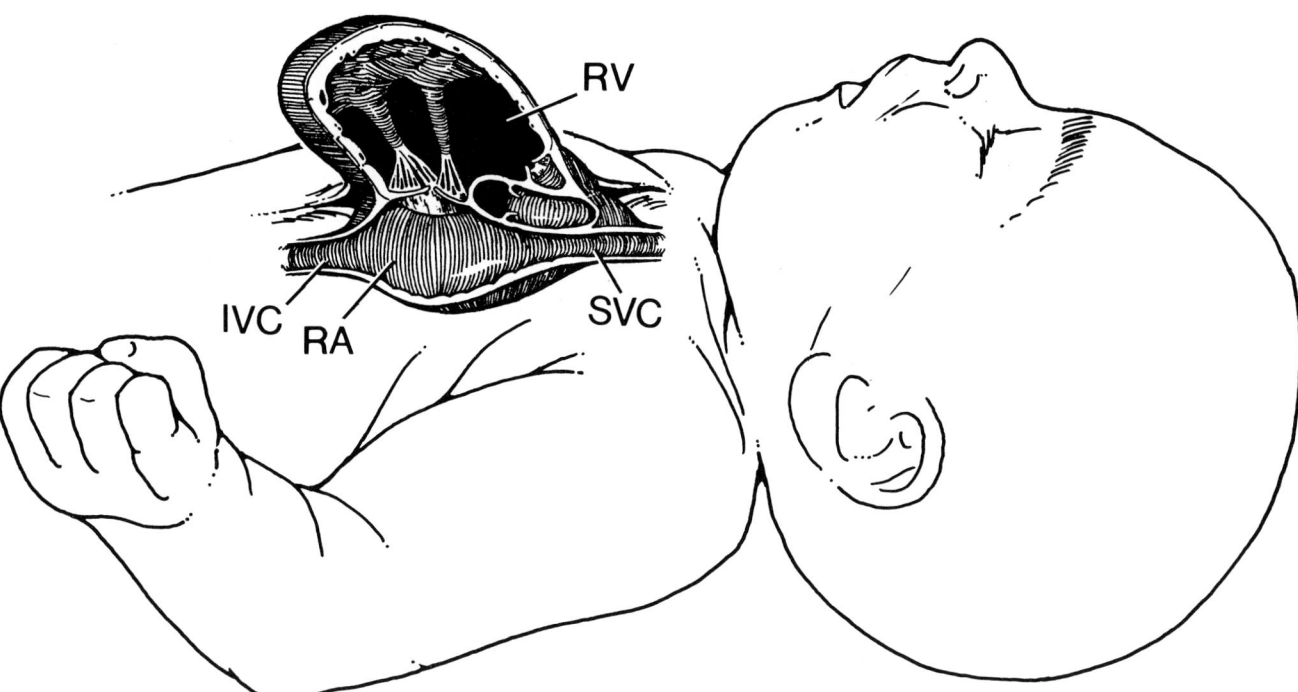

Fig. 4-26. Ectopia cordis. The fetal heart may be incompletely enclosed within the chest wall. RV = right ventricle; IVC = inferior vena cava; SVC = superior vena cava; RA = right atrium.

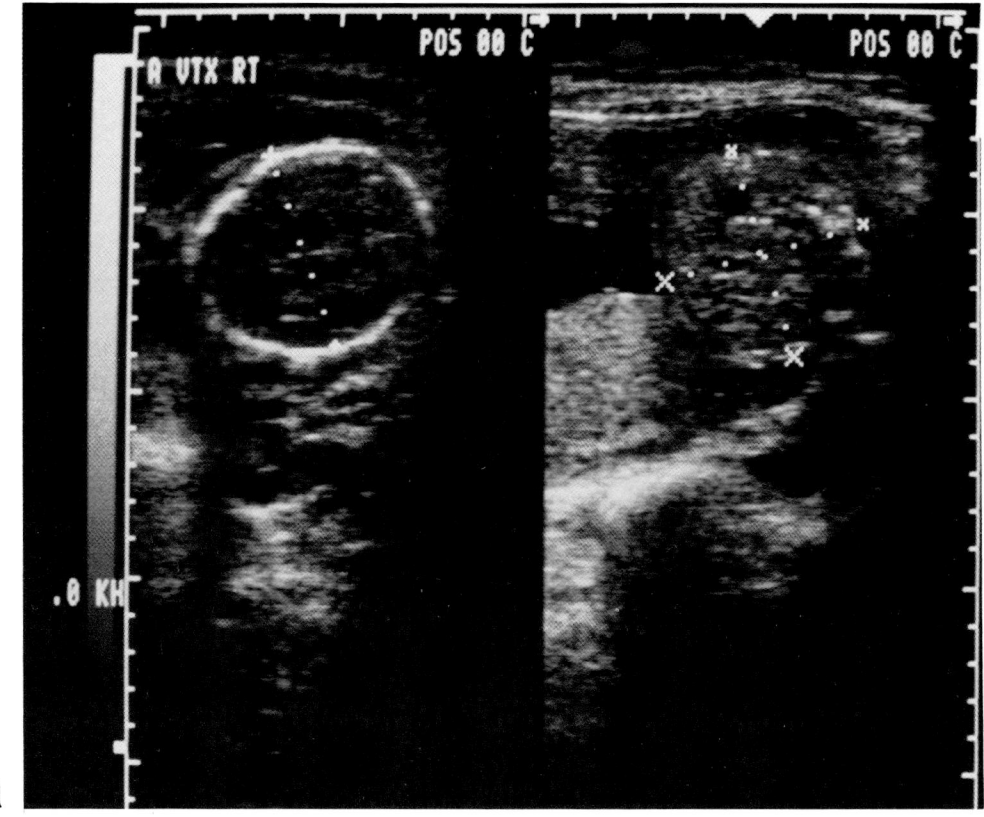

Fig. 4-27a-c. Twin–twin transfusion. Another circumstance in which a twin pregnancy can go awry is twin–twin transfusion; anastomoses of the placental arterial vasculature allow flow of blood between twins. Having too great a blood volume can be as lethal as too little. **a:** The donor twin (Hgb 7.6, weight 575 g); **b:** The recipient (Hgb 17.9, weight 470 g). Twin b shows evidence of growth retardation. **c:** Doppler ultrasound studies of the umbilical artery flows from both twins. The systolic-to-diastolic ratio for twin A is lower than would normally be seen at this gestational age. The systolic-to-diastolic ratio for twin B has reverse flow in diastole, which is an ominous sign. These twins were delivered within 10 days of the ultrasound study.

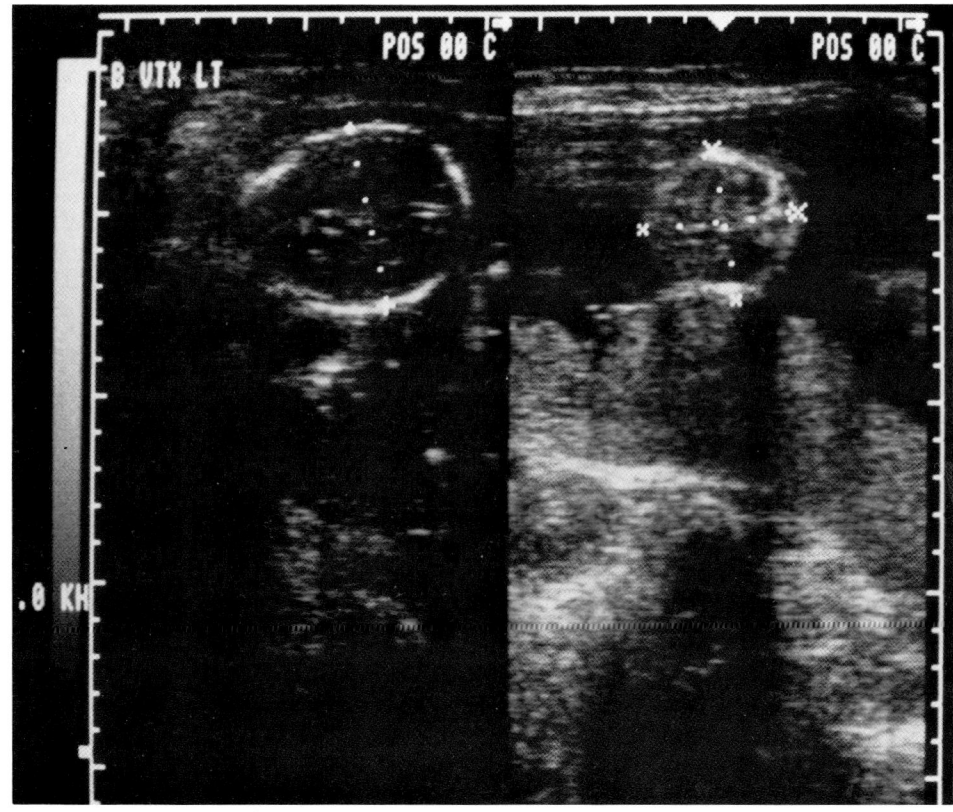

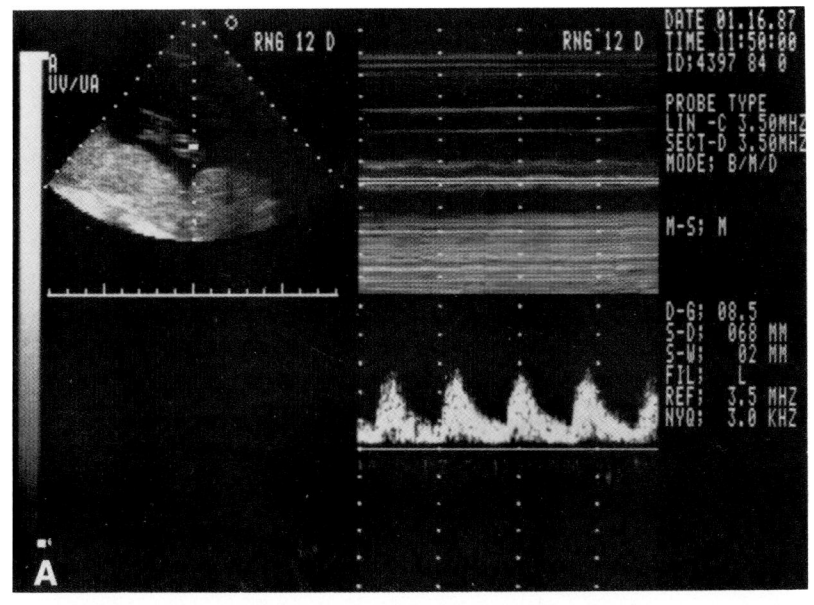
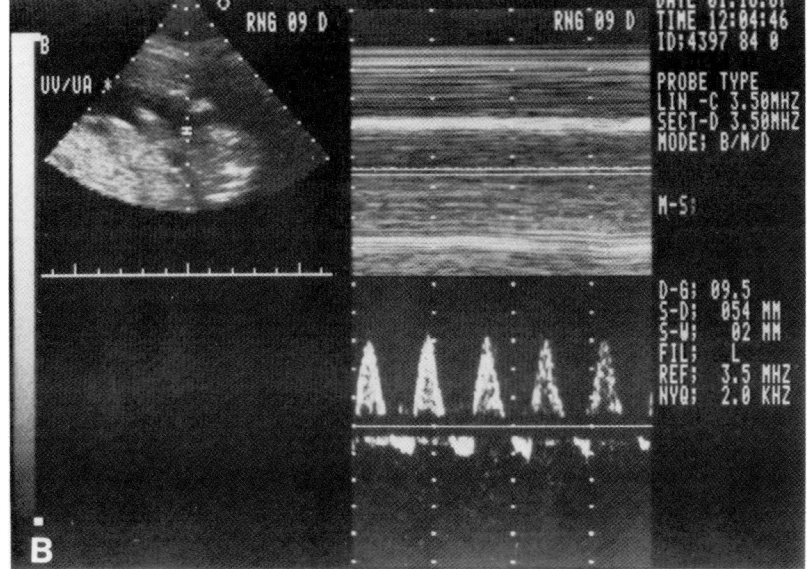

C

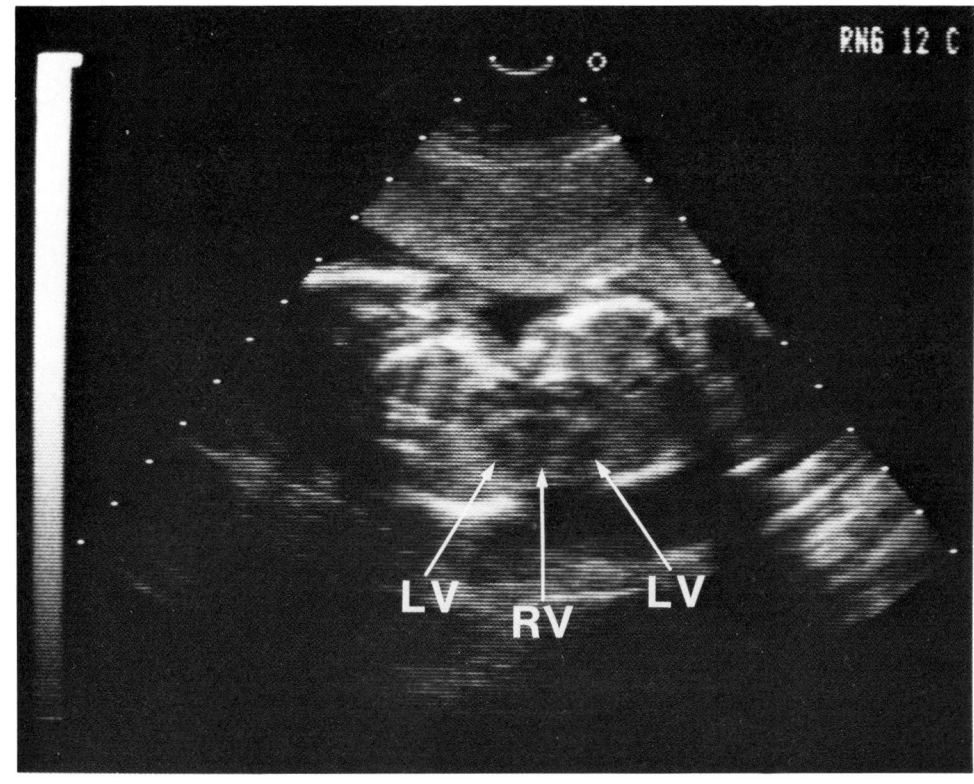

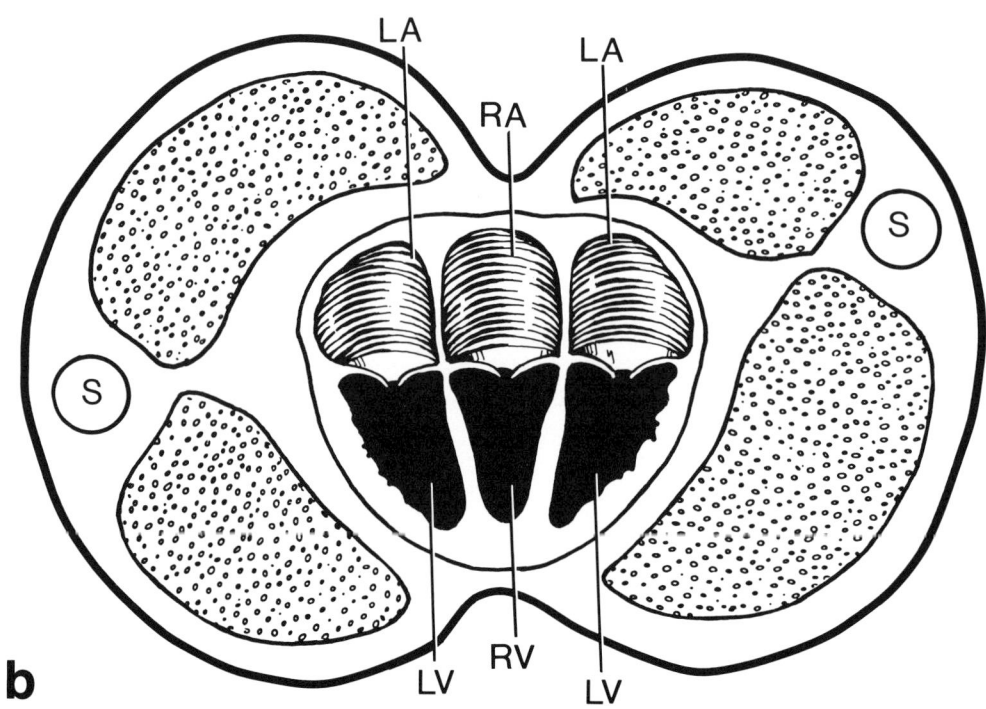

Fig. 4–28a,b. Thoracopagus. The mother of these twins conjoined at the sternum was referred at 19 weeks for a second opinion. The fetuses are joined from the upper thoraces to the lower abdomen. The livers and hearts are shared. In this view of the fetal thoraces, each fetus has a left ventricle (LV), but they share a common right ventricle (RV). LA = left atrium; RA = right atrium; S = spine.

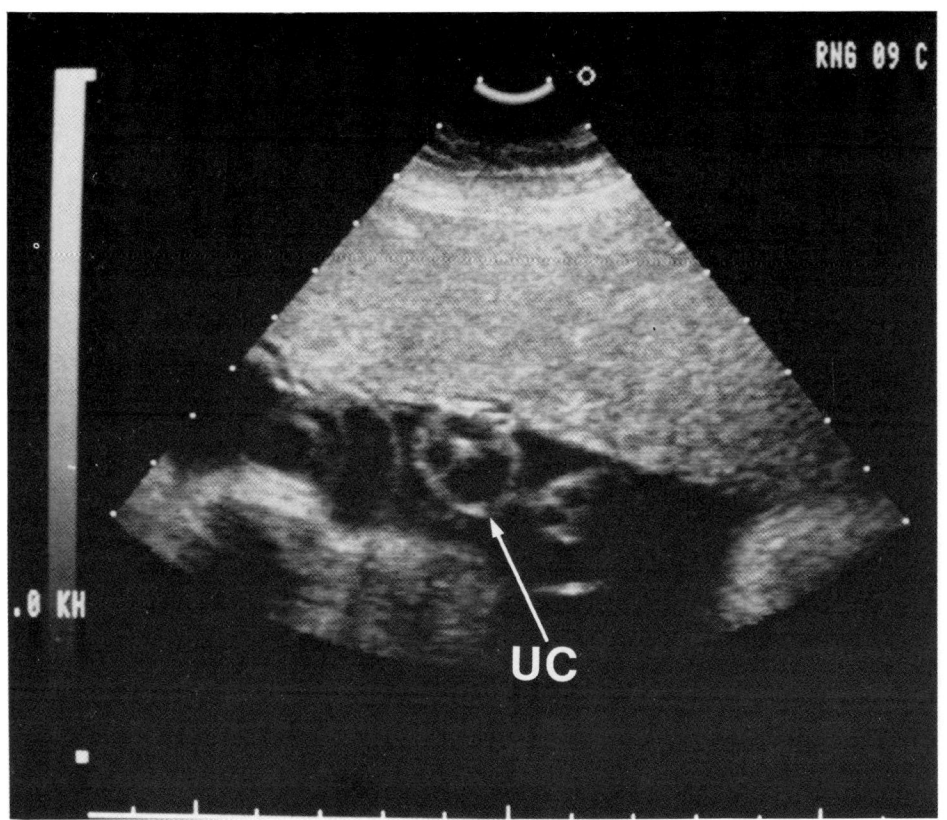

Fig. 4-29a. This is a cross section of a normal three-vessel cord (UC). The larger circular structure is the vein above which are seen the two arteries.

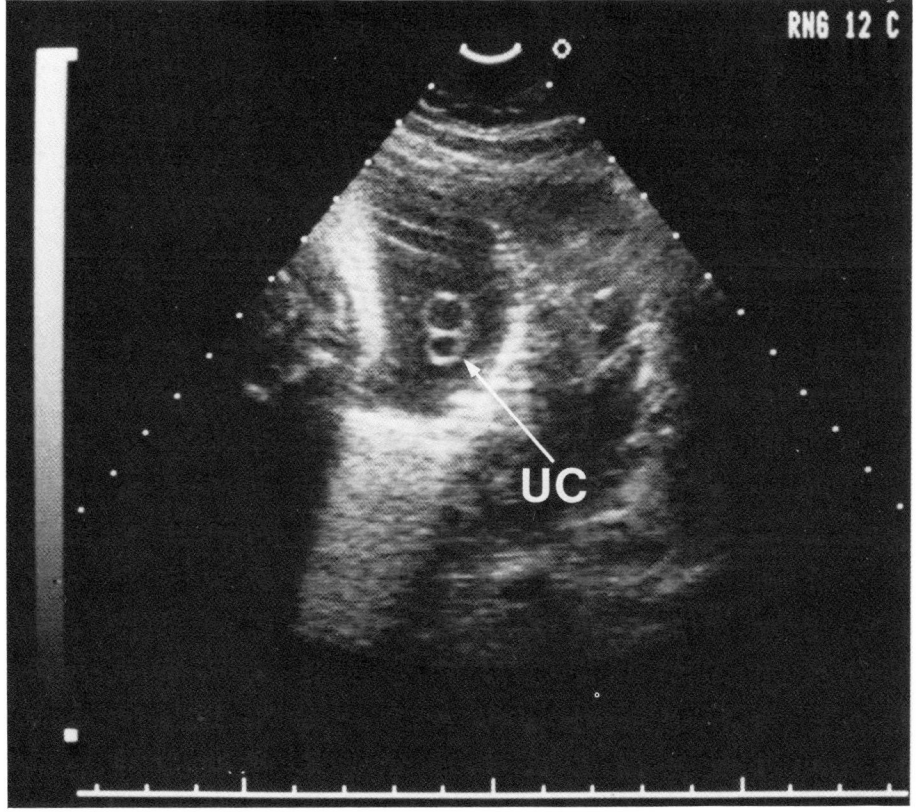

Fig. 4-29b. This two-vessel cord (UC) with its single umbilical artery situated posterior to the vein, gives a warning sign that the fetus should be carefully examined, since there is a higher probability of anomalies.

5

M-Mode Echocardiography

M-mode echocardiography utilizes detection of motion through time as a method by which to document cardiac activity. A cursor is placed across the heart, usually directed by two-dimensional echocardiography. An image, which records the motion detected by the cursor over time, is produced (Fig. 5–1).

The primary application of M-mode echocardiography in fetal examinations in the past was to document fetal cardiac activity. In adult and pediatric work, a pattern was established of imaging a continuum from the apex of the heart, across the mitral valve, and into the ascending aorta and atria. These examinations focused primarily on the left ventricle, since the right ventricle was more difficult to visualize, and the left ventricle tended to be most important in overall cardiac assessment. Because the fetal position is not always predictable or reproducible, this particular pattern of scanning is not usually possible in the fetus. Both the right and the left ventricle must be carefully evaluated in the fetus.

Applications of M-mode echocardiography to the fetal heart are summarized in Table 5–1. M-mode is very useful in establishing the type of arrhythmia present in fetuses with abnormal heart rhythms (Fig. 5–2). This is done by placing the cursor so that it crosses a structure that moves with the atrial contraction (atrial wall, atrioventricular valve leaflet) and a structure that moves with ventricular contraction (ventricular wall, semilunar valve leaflet). In this manner, the relation of atrial and ventric-

TABLE 5–1. Uses of M-Mode Echocardiography

Establish type of arrhythmia
   Premature contractions
   Tachyarrhythmias
   Complete heart block
Measure ventricular sizes
   Valve sizes
   Aortic size
Calculate fractional shortening
Document pericardial effusion
Document fetal cardiac activity

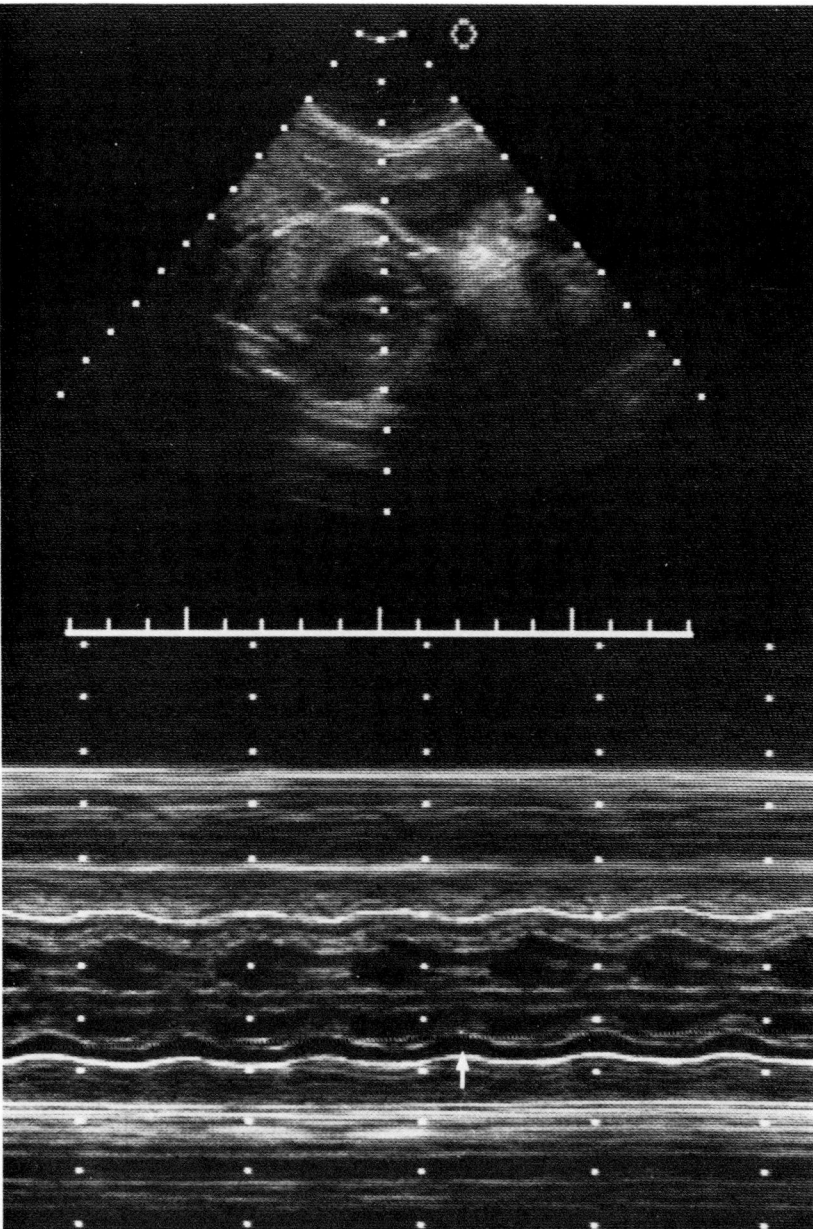

Fig. 5-1. Two-dimensional and M-mode echocardiogram in a fetus with a pericardial effusion. The cursor is placed across both ventricles simultaneously (right ventricle is above left ventricle). Arrow points to fluid in the pericardial space. This fetus had severe growth retardation.

ular contraction can be documented (Figs. 5-2 to 5-4 and Chapter 7). Premature atrial contractions (Fig. 5-2), both conducted and nonconducted, supraventricular tachycardia, including atrial fibrillation/flutter (Fig. 5-3) and paroxysmal atrial tachycardia, and complete heart block (Fig. 5-4) can be identified using this technique.

M-mode echocardiography has been used by several investigators [1,2] to measure ventricular sizes and aortic size. This is done by placing the cursor simultaneously across both ventricles. This view is also used to calculate fractional shortening, which is an index of ventricular function. Measurements can be taken during diastole and systole. Diastole occurs when ventricular walls are widest apart and atrioventricular valves are open.

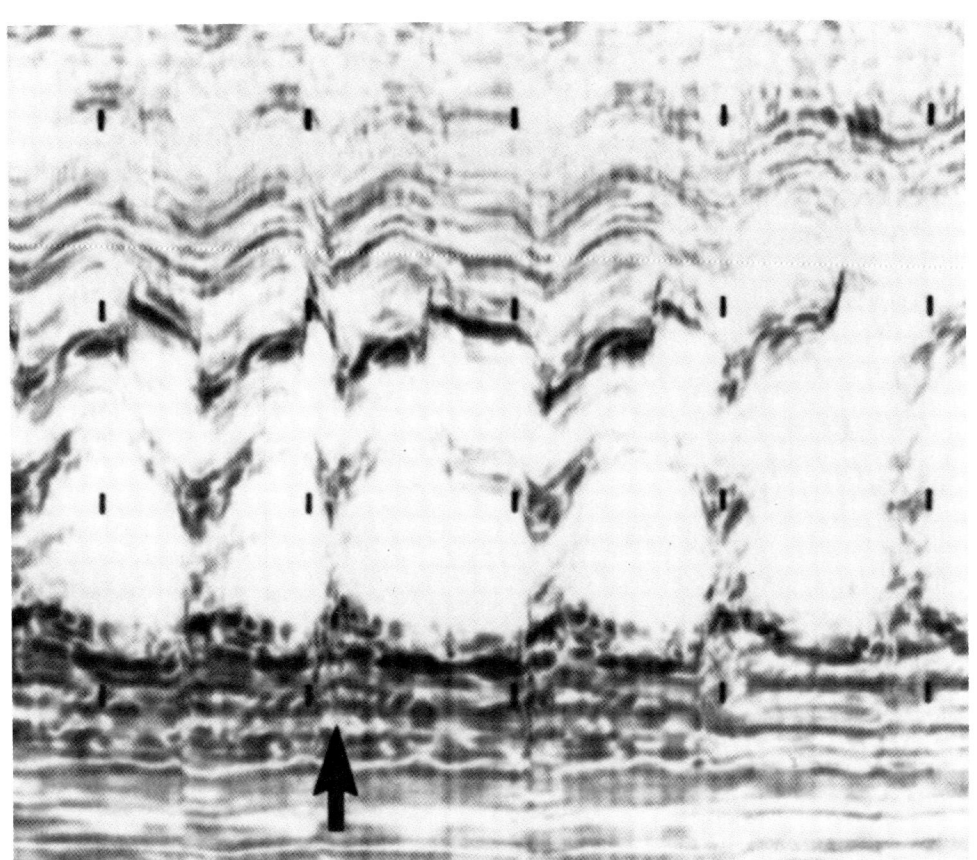

Fig. 5-2. M-mode echocardiography during a premature atrial contraction in a fetus. Arrow points to a premature contraction of the right atrial wall. The premature atrial beat is followed by a pause, with prolonged opening of the mitral valve and subsequent atrial and ventricular wall movement.

Systole occurs when ventricular walls are closest together and atrioventricular valves are closed. The formula for fractional shortening is (D − S)/D × 100. Fractional shortening ranges from 32% to 33% [1]. Using fractional shortening information in the fetus with premature atrial contractions, it has been possible to prove that postextrasystolic potentiation occurs in the human fetus [3]. Comparisons of aortic diameter to left atrial size have also been performed. The technique can be used to establish the presence of tetralogy of Fallot, since the aorta is enlarged [1]. Ventricular septal and wall hypertrophy may be seen using M-mode echocardiography (Fig. 5-5). These conditions may occur with maternal diabetes or with chronic abnormalities of blood flow. Chamber enlargement may be determined by diameter measurements obtained with M-mode echocardiography. Comparisons of measurements with those of other investigators [1,2] may help establish the degree of abnormality present.

M-mode echocardiography is also useful to establish the presence of a pericardial effusion (Fig. 5-1). Fluid can be seen between the heart and the pericardial sac. This amount of fluid is not normally present and may accompany congestive heart failure. M-mode measurements of cardiac valves may be used in calculations of volume flow in the fetus. Finally, images generated using M-mode echocardiography may be used simply to document fetal cardiac activity.

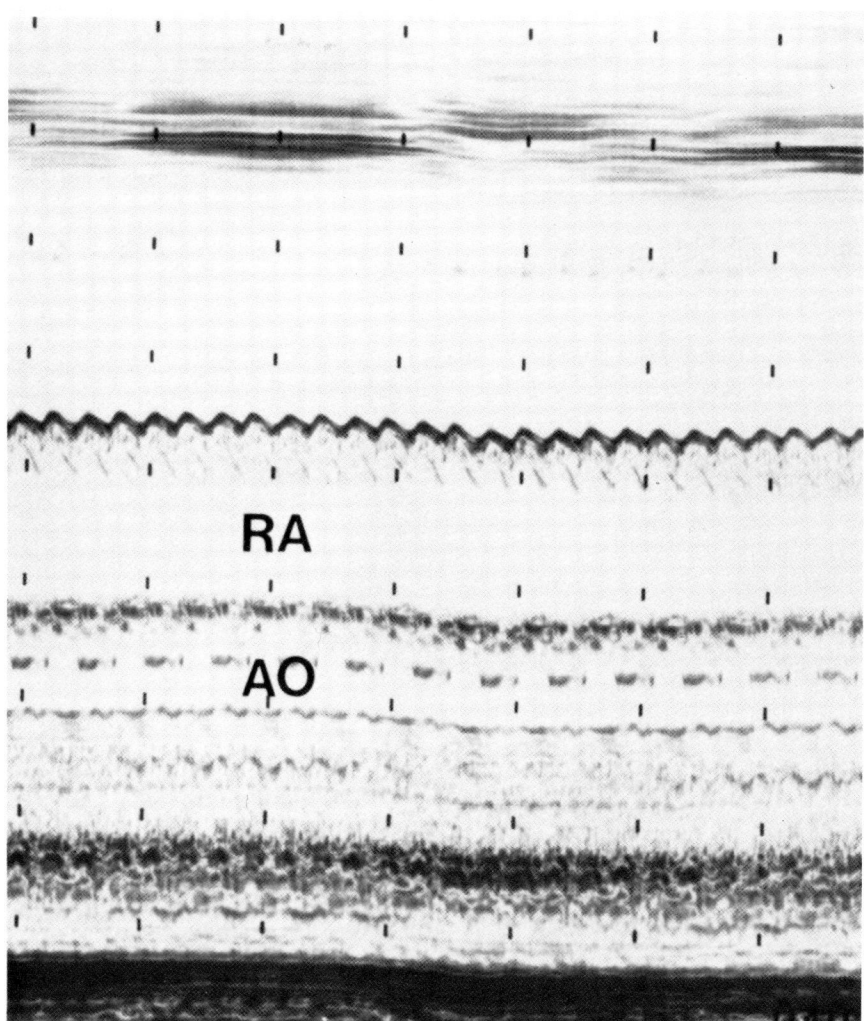

Fig. 5-3. M-mode echocardiogram from a fetus with pleural effusions and atrial flutter with 2:1 block. Right atrial wall (RA) is moving at a rate of 440 bpm. Superior to the right atrial wall, a collection of fluid is seen. Inferior to the right atrium, the aorta (AO) is seen, with dashes corresponding to aortic valve leaflet closure during diastole (220 bpm).

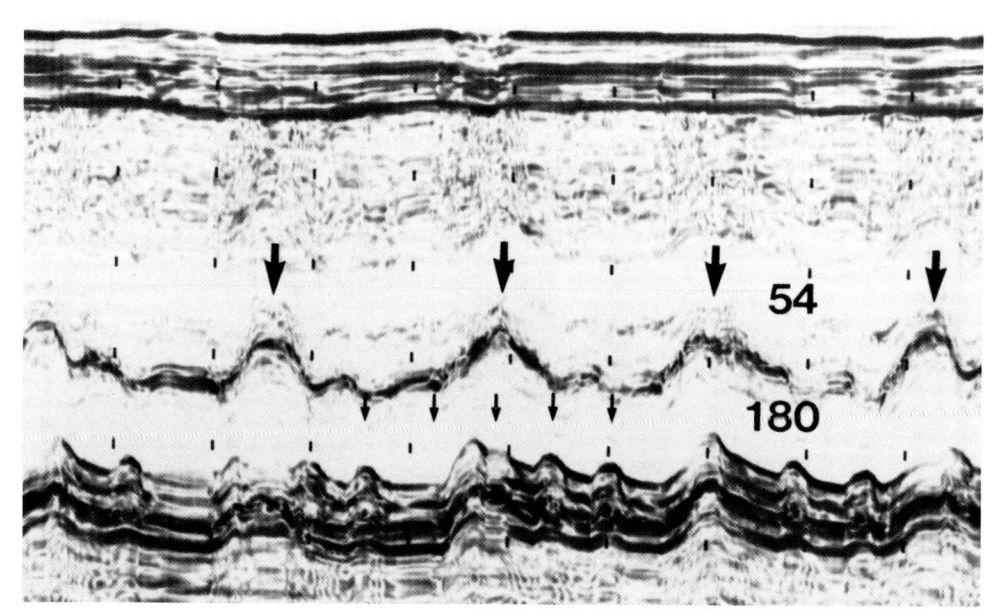

Fig. 5-4. M-mode echocardiogram from a fetus with complete heart block, atrial rate (small arrows) 180 bpm, ventricular rate (large arrows) 54 bpm. The mother, who was asymptomatic, was found to be ANA negative and anti-Ro antibody positive after fetal heart block was diagnosed. The fetus delivered vaginally at term and had a pacemaker placed after 48 hours.

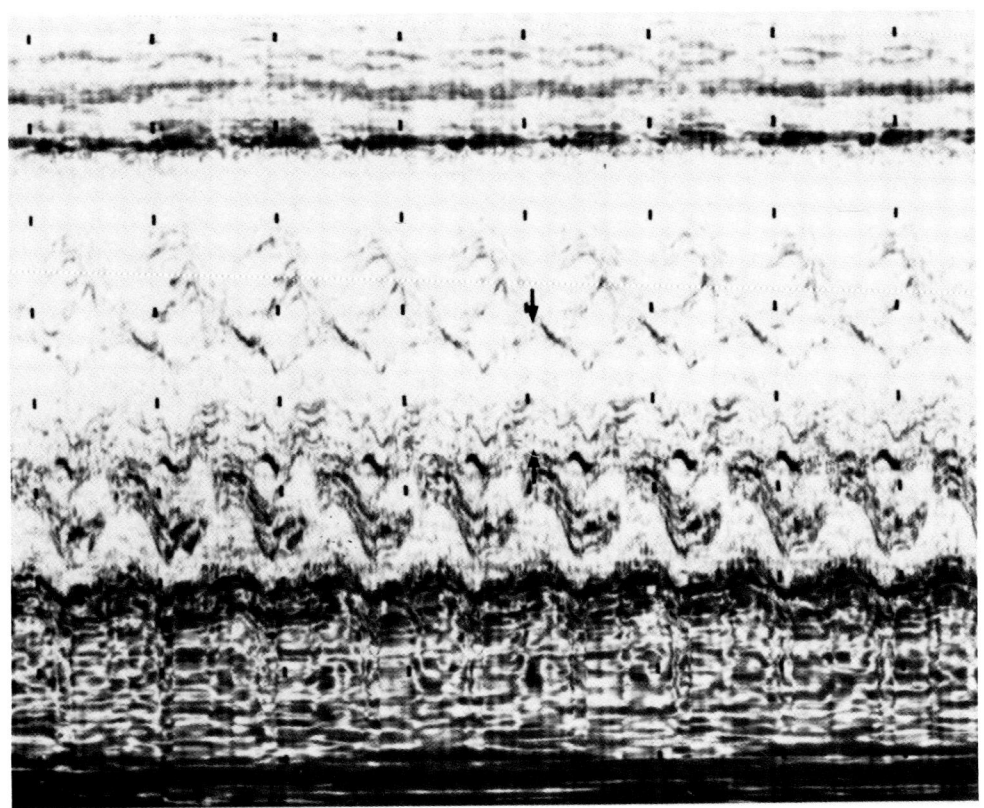

Fig. 5-5. M-mode echocardiogram from a fetus with septal hypertrophy (from a diabetic pregnancy). Arrows point to enlarged septum.

REFERENCES

1. DeVore GR: Cardiac Imaging. In Sabbagha RE (ed): Diagnostic Ultrasound, Ed. 2. Philadelphia: J. B. Lippincott Co., 1987.
2. Allan LD: Manual of Fetal Echocardiography. Boston: MTP, 1986.
3. Reed KL, Sahn DJ, Marx GR, et al.: Cardiac Doppler flows during fetal arrhythmias: Physiologic consequences. Obstet Gynecol 70:1–6, 1987.

6

Doppler Echocardiography

Doppler ultrasound investigations have been used to study fetal cardiovascular and umbilical–placental physiology (Table 6–1) [1]. It serves at present as an adjunctive technique in the establishment of fetal condition.

Doppler ultrasound techniques utilize the principle that energy (sound) reflected from a moving target (red blood cells) will change frequency in accordance with the direction and velocity of the target. This information can be translated into audible sound and a visualized tracing (Fig. 6–1). The relation of the speed recorded and the actual speed of the target varies with the cosine of the angle between the beam and the direction in which the target is moving. To establish the actual amount or volume of blood flow, measurement of the velocity of blood flow is necessary, along with measurement of the diameter of the vessel or valve through which the blood is flowing (from two-dimensional or M-mode examinations) [2].

Continuous-wave Doppler ultrasound techniques provide simultaneous detection of all vascular structures in the path of the beam. Pulsed Doppler ultrasound techniques measure the velocity at a more precise location. While equipment is available that provides only Doppler ultrasound information, many investigators prefer equipment that offers both two-dimensional imaging and a built-in or attached Doppler ultrasound unit.

TABLE 6–1. Applications of Doppler Ultrasound to the Human Fetus

Umbilical artery
Descending aorta
Umbilical vein
Inferior vena cava
Intracerebral artery
Maternal uterine arteries
Intracardiac valves
   Tricuspid
   Mitral
   Pulmonary
   Aorta

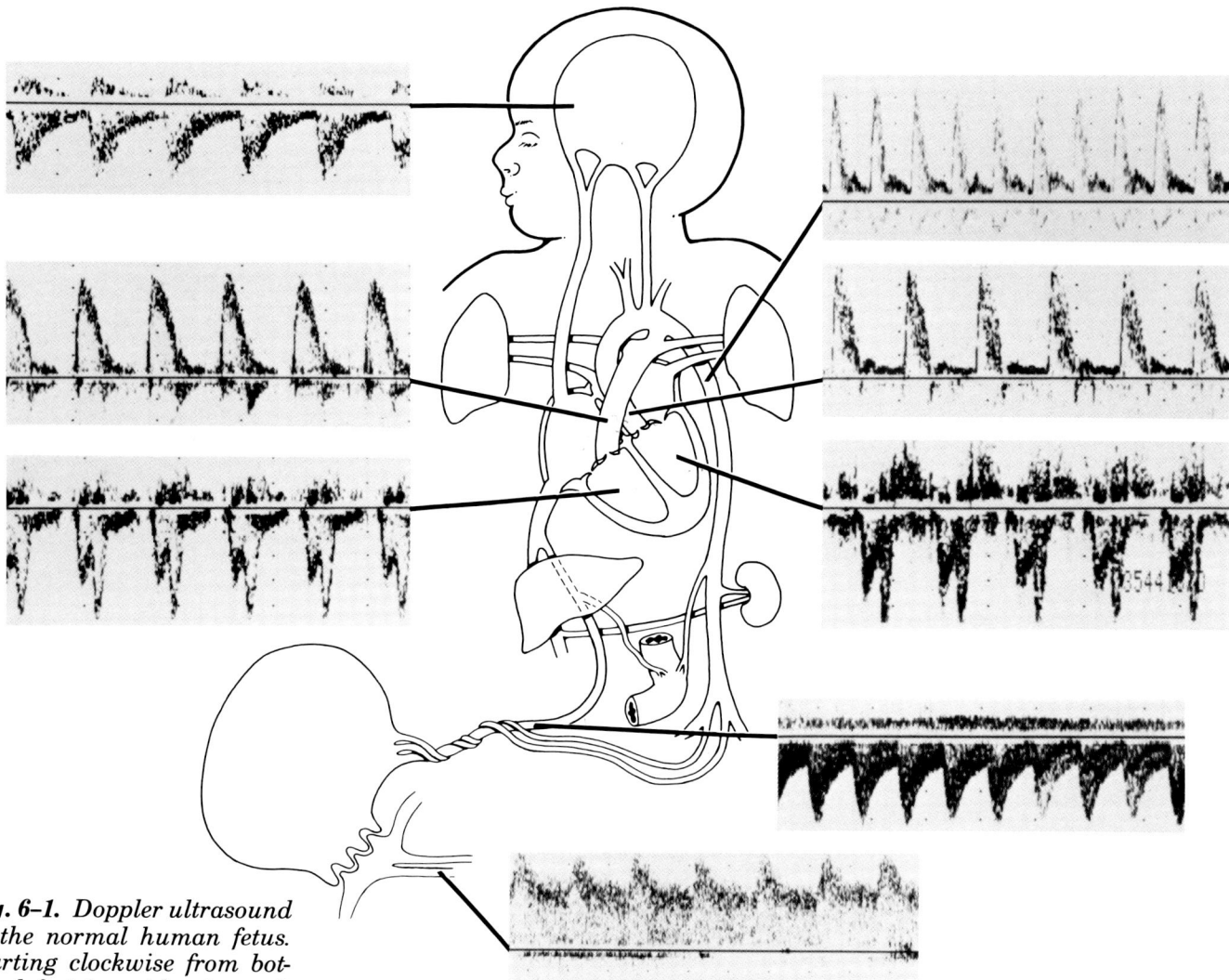

Fig. 6-1. Doppler ultrasound in the normal human fetus. Starting clockwise from bottom left: tricuspid valve, pulmonary valve, intracerebral arteries, descending aorta, aortic valve, mitral valve, umbilical artery and vein, and maternal vessels. (Adapted from Reed, 1987, with permission.)

Umbilical artery investigations have used both continuous-wave and pulsed Doppler ultrasound techniques. It is difficult to know the exact direction of blood flow in the umbilical artery; therefore most techniques of umbilical artery blood flow measurements involve comparisons of systolic and diastolic flow. The most commonly used measurement at present is the S/D ratio [3,4]. Other techniques include the pulsatility index, Pourcelot index (resistance index), and the frequency index profile [Table 6-2].

Investigators have shown that the S/D ratio decreases with gestational age from 4.0 ± 0.8 at 20 weeks to 2.0 ± 0.4 at 40 weeks [3-5]. If the S/D ratio is high for gestational age, the fetus is more likely to be growth-retarded (Fig. 6-2).

Similar measurements have been made from the descending aorta [6]. Ratios of systolic to diastolic flow have been reported. The waveform has been digitized, and volume flow has been calculated.

The velocity of blood flow through the umbilical vein also has been examined using Doppler ultrasound techniques [7]. Volume flow measure-

TABLE 6-2. Calculations for Umbilical Artery Doppler Ultrasound

S/D ratio
Pulsatility index
Pourcelot (resistance) index
Frequency index profile

TABLE 6-3. Normal Intracardiac Doppler Values in the Human Fetus

Parameter	TV	MV	PA	AO
Max (cm/sec)	51 ± 4	47 ± 4	60 ± 4	70 ± 3
Mean (cm/sec)	12 ± 1	11 ± 1	16 ± 2	18 ± 2
Volume flow (ml/kg/min)	307 ± 30	232 ± 25	312 ± 11	250 ± 9

TV = tricuspid valve; MV = mitral valve; PA = pulmonary artery; AO = aorta; min = minute; Max = maximal velocity; mean = mean velocity.

ments have been made from the intra-abdominal portion of the umbilical vein, and the normal rate of flow is 110–120 ml/kg/min. The inferior vena cava has also been examined, and further work is ongoing.

Maternal pelvic arterial structures have been studied using Doppler ultrasound techniques. There appears to be a relationship between the proportional amount of diastolic flow and the development of intrauterine growth retardation (Fig. 6–2).

Intracerebral arteries also can be studied using pulsed Doppler ultrasound techniques [8,9]. A normal ratio decreases from 8.0 to 4.0 during gestation. A lower ratio has been associated with intrauterine growth retardation.

Intracardiac studies have been performed since 1980. These consist of studies through the tricuspid, mitral, pulmonary, and aortic valves. Using two-dimensional ultrasound guidance, the cursor is placed just beyond the valve leaflets. Tracings are obtained, and maximal (highest peak) and mean (time–velocity integral area divided by cardiac cycle time) are derived from the strip chart recordings. Volume flow can be calculated when valve diameters are obtained. Ratios of peak velocity during late diastole (A) to peak velocity during early diastole (E) have been examined.

Using intracardiac Doppler ultrasound measurements, we have determined that 1) the fetal right heart volume flow is greater than left heart volume flow by a ratio of 1.3:1 (Table 6–3) [10]; 2) the A/E ratio is greater than one; this ratio decreased with gestational age, suggesting that the fetal heart is less compliant than the infant or adult heart and that fetal cardiac function changes during gestation [11]; 3) postextrasystolic potentiation and the Frank-Starling mechanism are operative in the human fetus [12]; and 4) cardiac function changes at birth [13].

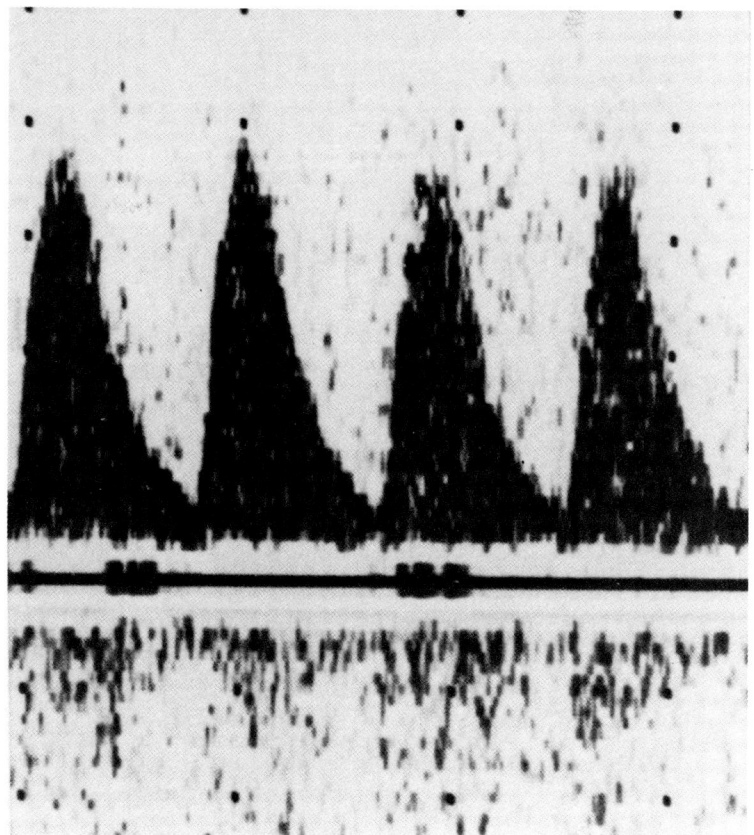

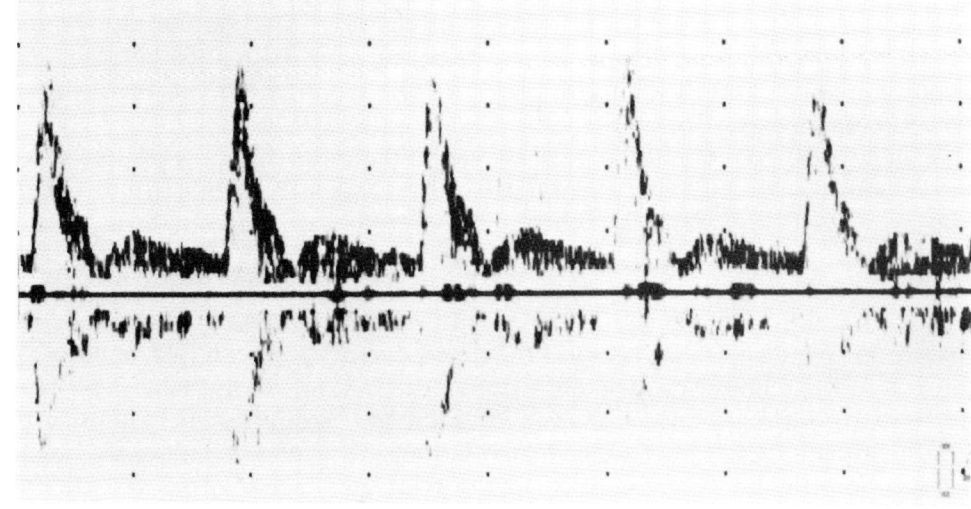

Fig. 6-2. Abnormal Doppler ultrasound tracings (**a**) from the umbilical artery of a fetus with growth retardation and Down syndrome (S/D ratio 6.2) and (**b**) from the maternal parauterine arteries of a woman with hypertension (compare with Fig. 6-1).

The major application of Doppler intracardiac studies from a clinical standpoint has been to confirm the presence of congenital cardiac anomalies. Examples include tetralogy of Fallot, pulmonary atresia, hypoplastic left heart (Fig. 6-3), atrioventricular canal defect, tricuspid atresia, double-outlet right ventricle, and Ebstein's anomaly (Table 6-4) [14].

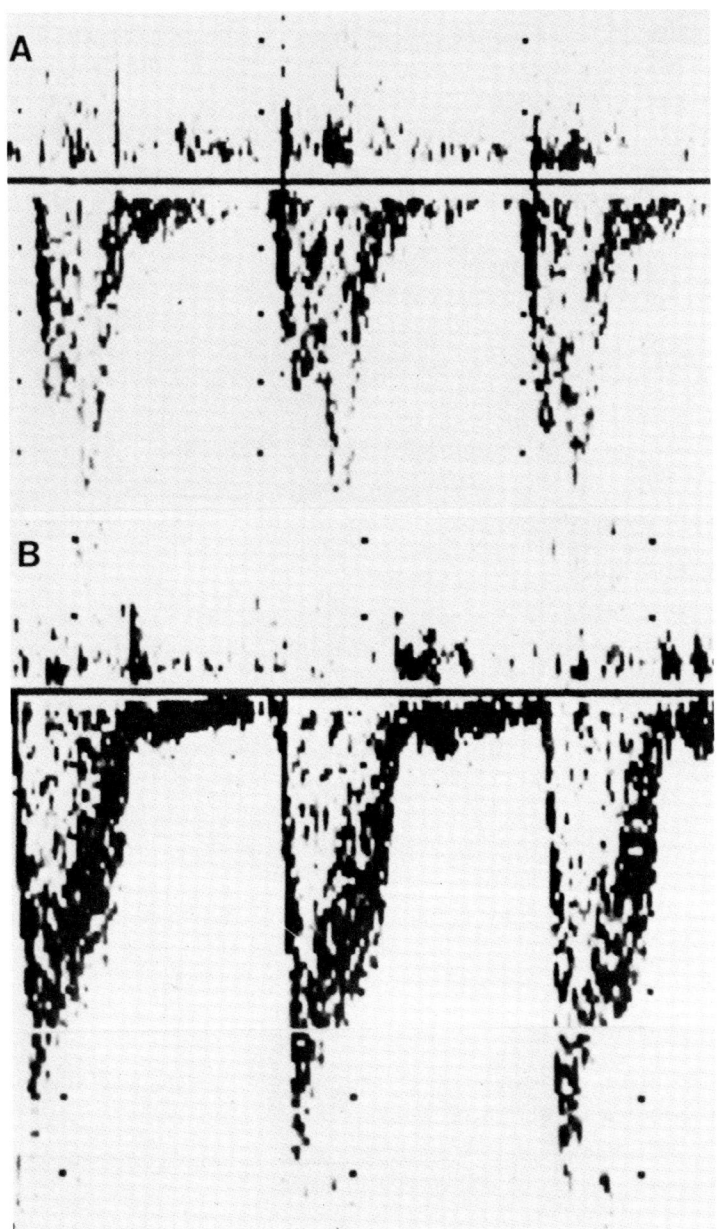

Fig. 6-3. A: Tricuspid valve; B: pulmonary artery Doppler ultrasound flow velocity tracings from a fetus with hypoplastic left heart syndrome. Mean Doppler velocities (tricuspid valve 19 cm/sec, pulmonary artery 29 cm/sec) are elevated compared to normal. Tracings could not be obtained from the mitral valve or the aorta.

TABLE 6–4. Changes in Doppler Blood Flow Velocities With Congenital Heart Disease

Abnormality	TV	MV	PA	AO
Hypoplastic left heart	↑V		↑	
Tetralogy of Fallot	=	=	↓	↑
Double-outlet right ventricle	=	=	=	=
Tricuspid atresia/TGV		↑	=	=
Pulmonary atresia	↑V	=		↑
Atrioventricular canal	↑V	↑V	↓	↑
Ebstein's anomaly	↑V	=	↓	=

TV = tricuspid valve; MV = mitral valve; PA = pulmonary artery; AO = aorta; TGV = transposition of the great vessels; V = regurgitation.

Doppler ultrasound studies can be used to demonstrate stenotic valves, insufficient valves, and abnormal shunts [2]. Color Doppler ultrasound studies are also useful (see Chapter 8).

In summary, the use of Doppler ultrasound has added a further dimension to the assessment of the fetal cardiovascular system and fetal well-being. Doppler ultrasound investigations are still in an evolutionary stage.

REFERENCES

1. Reed KL: Fetal and neonatal cardiac assessment with Doppler. Semin Perinatol 11:347–356, 1987.
2. Hatle L, Angelsen B: Doppler Ultrasound in Cardiology. Philadelphia: Lea & Febiger, 1985.
3. Schulman H, Fleischer A, Stern W, Farmakides G, Jagani N, Blattner P: Umbilical velocity wave ratios in human pregnancy. Am J Obstet Gynecol 148:985–990, 1984.
4. Trudinger BJ, Giles WB, Cook MB: Flow velocity waveforms in the maternal uteroplacental and fetal umbilical placental circulation. Am J Obstet Gynecol 152:155–163, 1985.
5. Reed KL, Anderson CF, Shenker L: Doppler studies of umbilical and uteroplacental vasculature in human pregnancy. Presented at the American Institute of Ultrasound in Medicine, New Orleans, October 6–9, 1987.
6. Griffin D, Bilardo K, Masini L, et al: Doppler blood flow waveforms in the descending thoracic aorta of the human fetus. Br J Obstet Gynaecol 91:997–1006, 1984.
7. Gill RW, Warren PS, Garrett WJ, et al: Umbilical venous flow in normal and complicated pregnancy. Ultrasound Med Biol 10:349–363, 1984.
8. Wladimiroff JW, Tonge HM, Stewart P: Doppler ultrasound assessment of cerebral blood flow in the human fetus. Br J Obstet Gynaecol 93:471–475, 1986.
9. Arduini D, Rizzo G, Romanini C, Mancuso, S: Fetal blood flow velocity waveforms as predictors of growth retardation. Obstet Gynecol 70:7, 1987.
10. Reed KL, Meijboom EJ, Scagnelli SA, et al: Cardiac Doppler flow velocities in human fetuses. Circulation 73:41–46, 1986.
11. Reed KL, Sahn DJ, Scagnelli S, et al: Doppler echocardiographic studies of diastolic function in the human fetal heart: Changes during gestation. J Am Coll Cardiol 8:391–395, 1986.
12. Reed KL, Sahn DJ, Marx GR, et al: Cardiac Doppler flows during fetal arrhythmias: Physiologic consequences. Obstet Gynecol 70:1–6, 1987.
13. Wilson N, Reed KL, Allen HD, et al: Doppler echocardiographic observations of pulmonary and transvalvular velocity changes after birth and during the early neonatal period. Am Heart J 113:750–758, 1987.
14. Shenker L, Reed KL, Marx GR, et al: Fetal cardiac Doppler flow studies in the prenatal diagnosis of heart disease. Am J Obstet Gynecol (in press).

7

Fetal Cardiac Arrhythmias

Arrhythmias vary in clinical significance; it is important to make as accurate a diagnosis as possible whenever an irregular, abnormally slow, or rapid rate is found. Echocardiography provides the most consistently accurate means not only to confirm the presence of an arrhythmia but to specifically identify the type of arrhythmia and provide information about its effect on fetal well-being.

The most useful ultrasound examinations for fetal cardiac arrhythmias are two-dimensional (for anatomy) and M-mode. The M-mode is particularly useful if the M-mode cursor is positioned such that it intersects both an atrial wall and a ventricular wall, recording simultaneous motion of both chambers (Fig. 7–1). Observation of atrioventricular or semilunar valve motion is also helpful. Doppler flow velocity studies provide additional information about the effects of the arrhythmia on cardiac function.

Since most arrhythmias are first detected by listening to the fetal heart, a classification based on auscultatory findings is helpful (Table 7–1). On rare occasions, a fetal cardiac arrhythmia may be detected when antepar-

TABLE 7-1. Classification of Arrhythmias Based on Auscultatory Findings

Irregular rhythms
  Premature atrial contractions
    Conducted
    Nonconducted (blocked)
    Combination of conducted and nonconducted
  Premature ventricular contractions
  Tachyarrhythmias with atrioventricular block

Rapid rates (> 180 bpm)
  Sinus tachycardia
  Atrial tachycardia
  Atrial flutter/fibrillation

Slow rates (< 110 bpm)
  Nonconducted (blocked) atrial premature contractions
  Complete heart block
  Sinus bradycardia

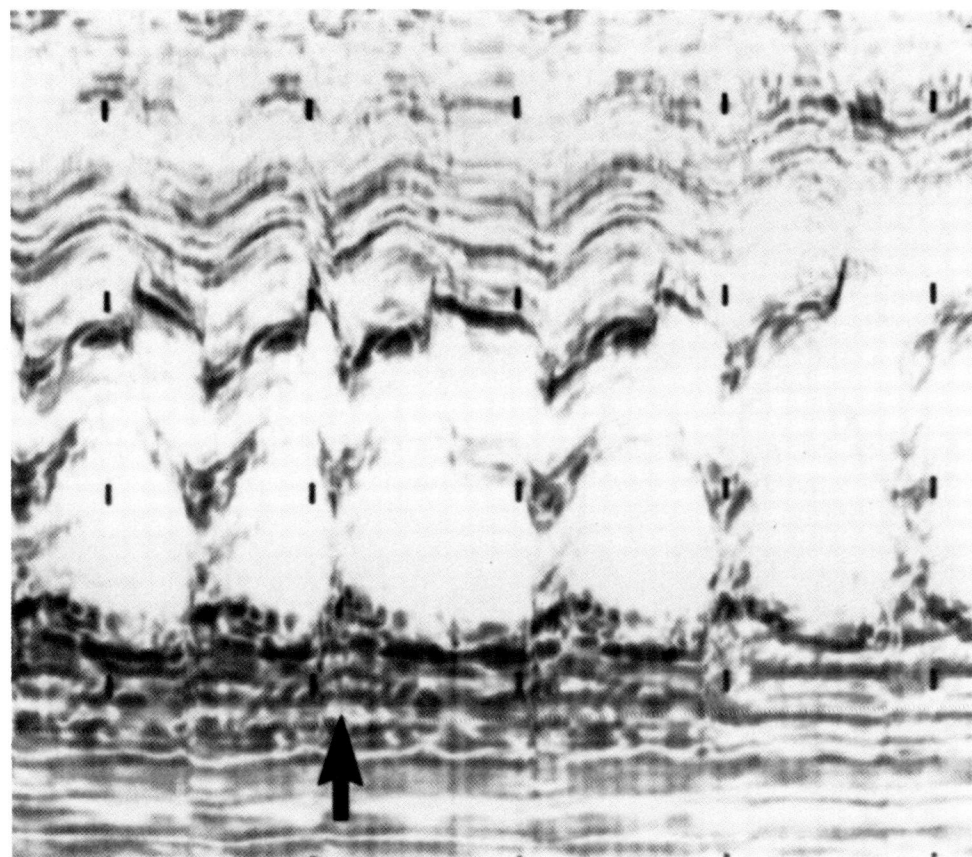

Fig. 7-1. M-mode echocardiography during a conducted premature atrial contraction in a fetus. Arrow points to a premature contraction of the right atrial wall. The premature atrial beat is followed by a pause, with prolonged opening of the mitral valve and subsequent atrial and ventricular wall movement.

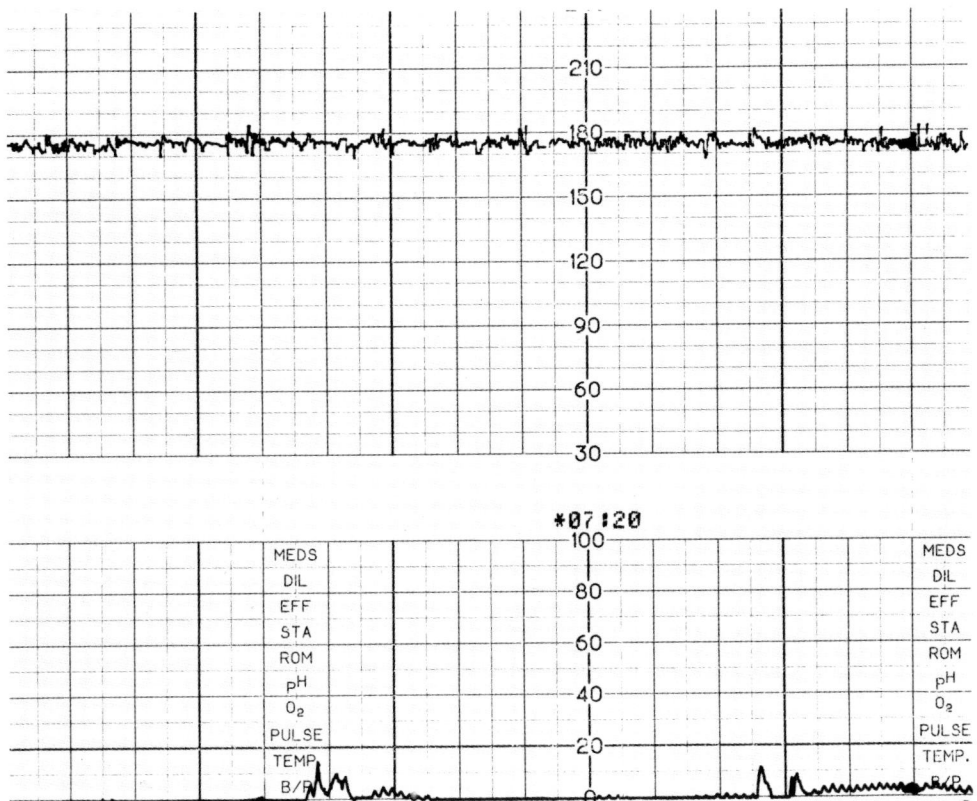

Fig. 7-2. Fetal monitoring strip from a fetus with tachycardia (175 bpm). Note decrease in variability. Figure 7-12 shows the M-mode echocardiogram recorded when this fetus was examined with ultrasound.

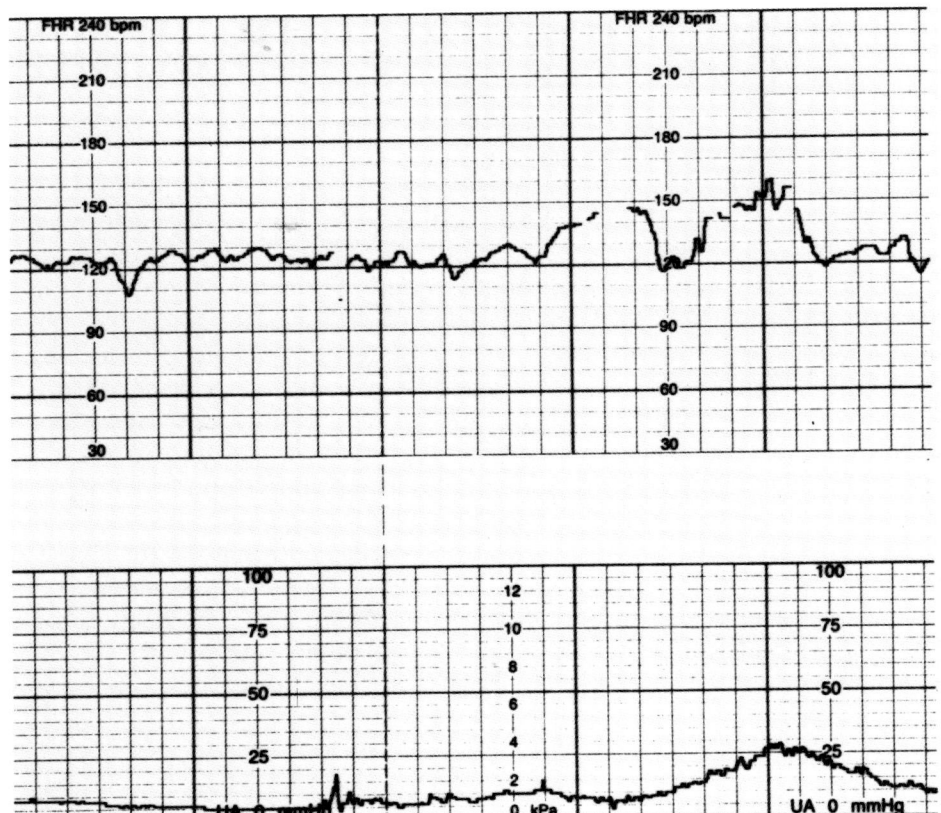

Fig. 7-3. Fetal monitoring strip from the same fetus after conversion of atrial flutter to normal sinus rhythm (4 days after the previous study). Note the increase in heart rate variability and the normal appearance of the strip compared to Figure 7-2.

tum fetal cardiac monitoring during a non-stress test reveals a loss of short- and long-term heart rate variability. This can occur with atrial tachycardia or atrial flutter with a 2:1 or 3:1 atrioventricular block. (Figs. 7-2, 7-3).

Premature atrial contractions are the most frequently observed arrhythmia in the fetus (Figs. 7-1, 7-4 to 7-7) [1]. The atrial contractions may be conducted (Figs. 7-1, 7-4), nonconducted (Fig. 7-5), or a combination of conducted and nonconducted (Figs. 7-6, 7-7). During the prenatal course the premature contractions may be intermittent in occurrence. They may disappear during labor or during the first few days of life. They are usually well tolerated by the fetus and need no special treatment. Observation is indicated to identify the few instances in which the rhythm converts to atrial tachycardia.

Conducted or nonconducted premature atrial contractions can produce irregular fetal heart sounds. The major significance of this arrhythmia is that when nonconducted premature atrial contractions occur frequently, they produce fetal bradycardia, which may be mistaken for fetal distress, or for complete heart block. M-mode echocardiographic studies will differentiate among these diagnoses, by visualizing atrial wall, atrioventricular valve, and ventricular wall motion. The appearance of atrial wall motion occurring prematurely and not causing normal atrioventricular valve motion or resulting in a ventricular contraction is diagnostic of nonconducted atrial premature beats. Premature atrial contractions are infrequently accompanied by structural fetal cardiac disease. Doppler ultrasound studies of the umbilical artery (Fig. 7-7) will show a variety of systolic peak/diastolic trough ratios in the presence of an irregular heart rate and should be carefully interpreted in these cases, since the fetuses are usually healthy.

Premature ventricular contractions (Figs. 7-8, 7-9) are less frequently observed than premature atrial contractions and are rarely accompanied by structural cardiac diseases. Premature ventricular contractions can be distinguished from premature atrial contractions by M-mode echocardiography. The premature ventricular wall motion is not preceded by atrial wall motion and is usually followed by a longer pause than if the premature contraction arises in the atrium.

Atrial tachycardia (Figs. 7-10 to 7-12) is a clinically significant arrhythmia. If persistent, atrial tachycardia will lead to fetal cardiac failure manifested by fetal hydrops with pericardial and pleural effusions and ascites (Fig. 7-11). There may be atrial dilation and tricuspid valve insufficiency, which can be confirmed by Doppler flow velocity studies [2]. This arrhythmia is responsive to intrauterine medical therapy, which allows fetal improvement and prolongation of the pregnancy in indicated cases [3].

Complete heart block (Figs. 7-13 to 7-15) may be an indication of maternal connective tissue disease. Anti-Ro antibody is frequently present in maternal blood. Complete heart block may be accompanied by complex and often lethal structural heart disease [4].

Although the other arrhythmias are rarely complicated by structural heart disease, it is important that they be accurately diagnosed so that patients can be appropriately monitored and reassured. Prenatal diagnosis assures that the newborn will be delivered in an appropriate facility if early further diagnostic and therapeutic steps are indicated.

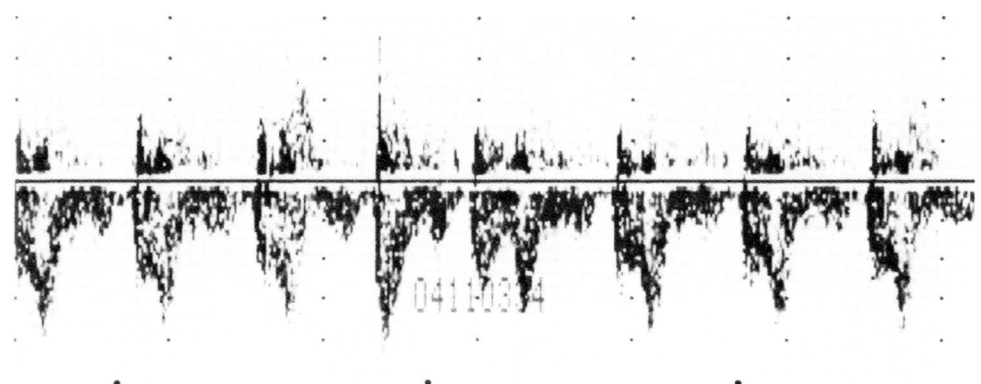

Fig. 7-4. *Doppler ultrasound tracing from the tricuspid valve of a fetus with conducted premature atrial contractions. The initial three waveforms and last three waveforms are normal; the premature beat (single peak) is early compared with the atrial peak of the preceding beat. The waveform following the premature beat is larger and longer than the normal beats.*

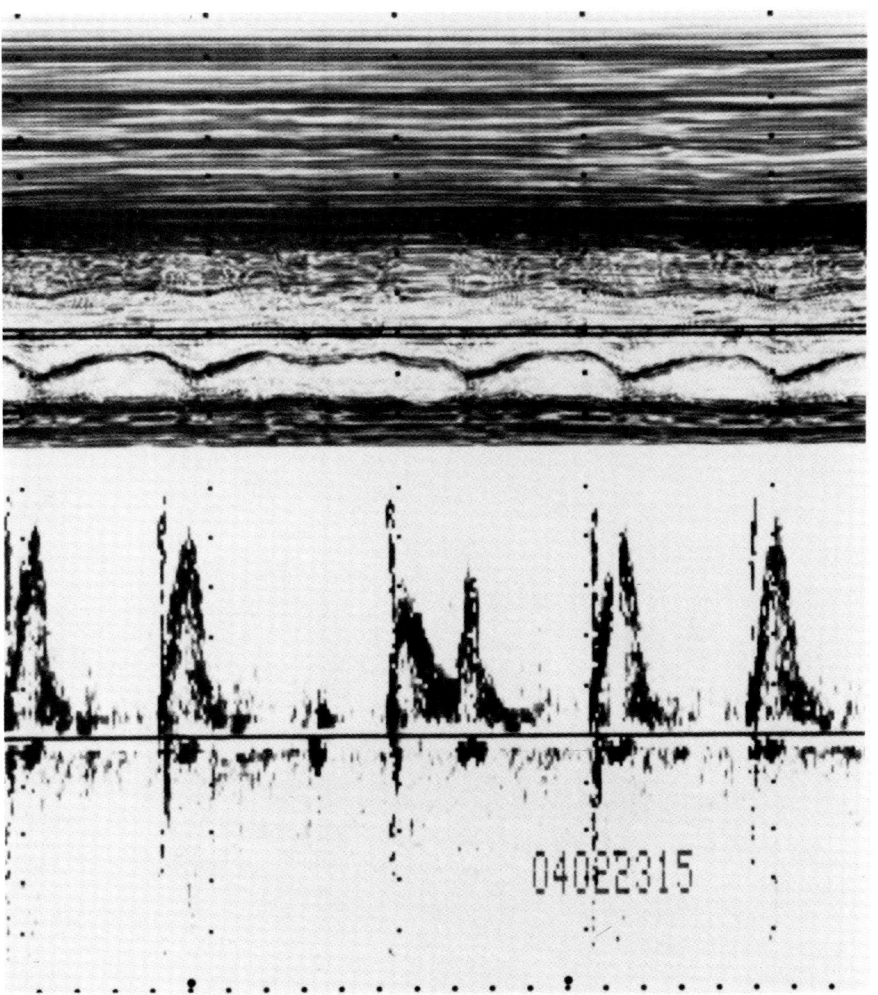

Fig. 7-5. *Doppler ultrasound tracing from a fetus with a nonconducted premature atrial contraction. Since the atrial beat is nonconducted, no flow occurs through the tricuspid valve during the contraction. Flow into the right ventricle during the pause following the premature beat is prolonged. The first two and last two waveforms on the strip appear normal.*

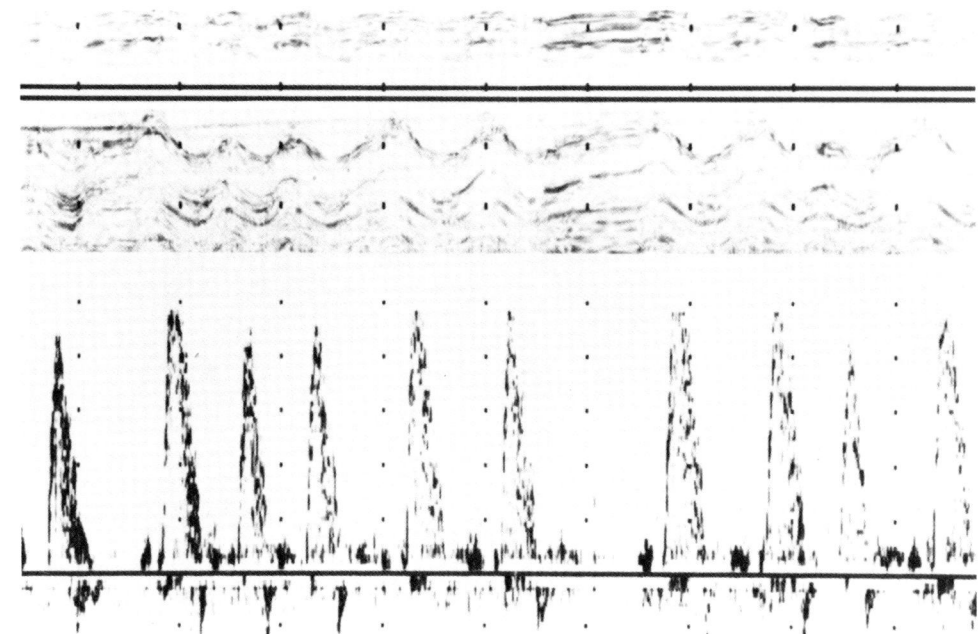

Fig. 7-6. M-mode and Doppler flow velocity tracing from a fetus with conducted and nonconducted premature atrial contractions. Flow is across the aortic valve. Conducted premature beats are the smallest waveforms; waveforms following conducted premature beats are larger; and waveforms following blocked premature beats are largest.

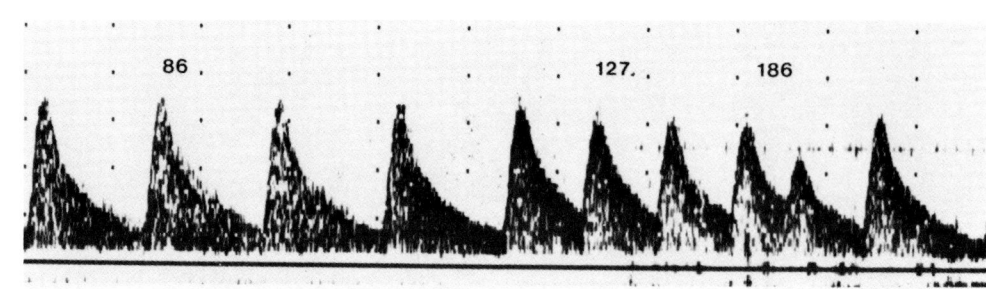

Fig. 7-7. Umbilical artery Doppler tracing from a fetus with conducted and nonconducted premature atrial contractions. Note the variation in systolic peaks and diastolic troughs, depending on the onset of systole and the duration of diastole. Heart rates are seen superior to tracing.

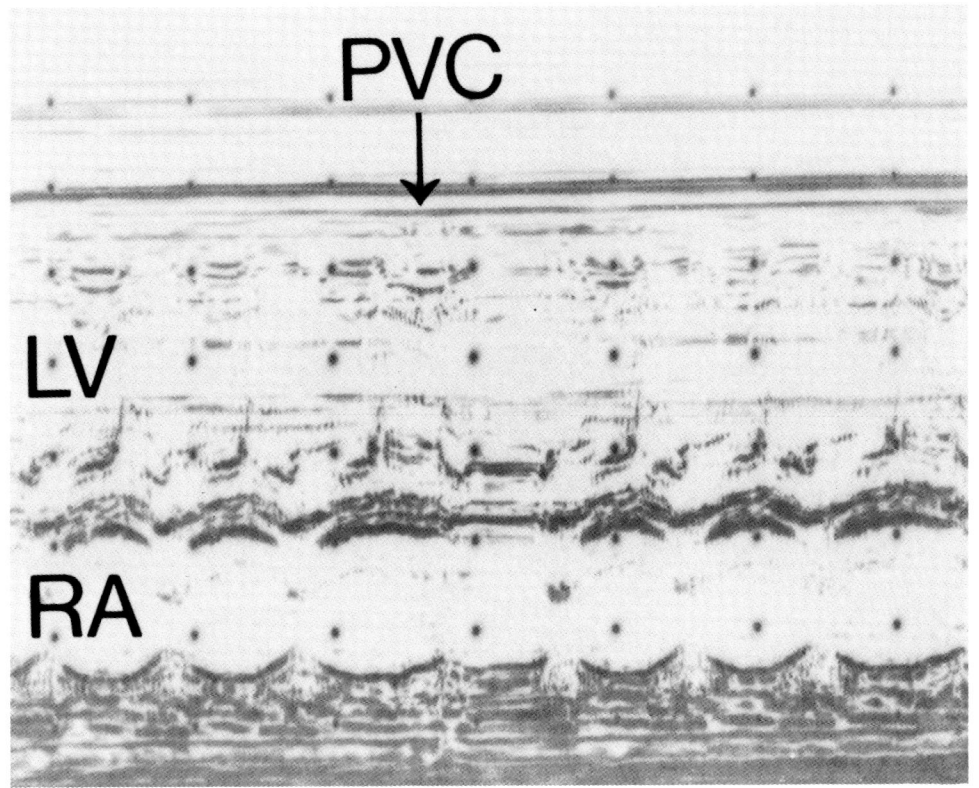

Fig. 7–8. M-mode echocardiogram in a fetus with premature ventricular contractions (PVC). Arrow points to premature ventricular wall contraction. LV = left ventricle; RA = right atrium.

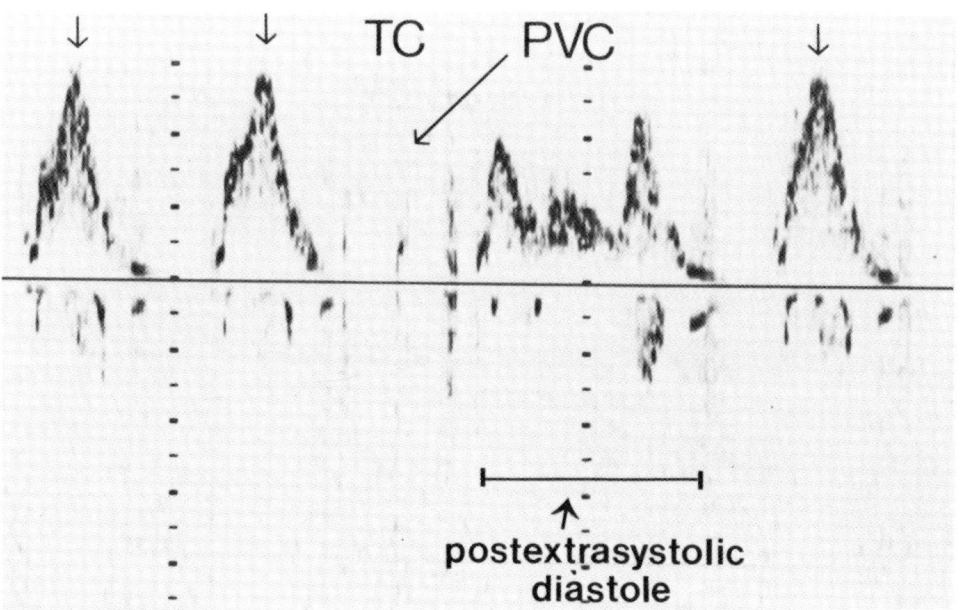

Fig. 7–9. Doppler flow velocity tracing of flow across the tricuspid valve (TC) in a fetus with premature ventricular contractions (PVC). Short arrows point to normal waveforms. No ventricular filling is seen during the PVC (long arrow). Flow following the premature beat is prolonged (postextrasystolic diastole).

Fig. 7-10. M-mode echocardiography from a fetus with intermittent supraventricular tachycardia, atrial bigeminy, and normal sinus rhythm. The strip begins with tachycardia (180 bpm) and ends with atrial bigeminy (90 bpm). Atrial wall is the upper dark line; valvular motion is seen in the center.

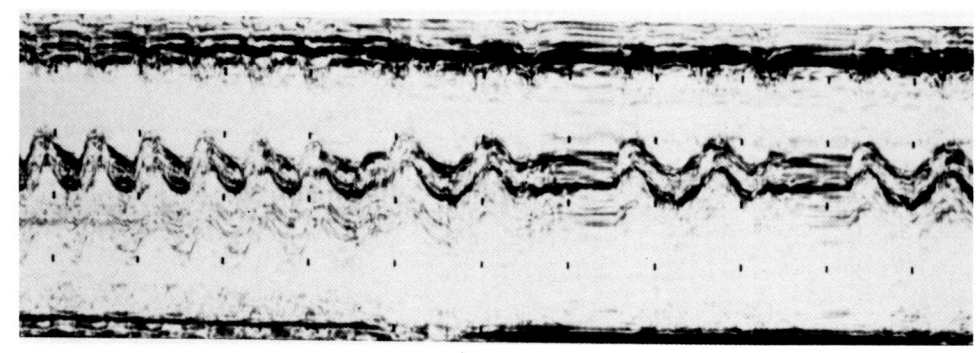

Fig. 7-11. M-mode echocardiogram from a fetus with pleural effusions and atrial flutter with 2:1 block. Right atrial wall (RA) is moving at a rate of 440 bpm. Superior to the right atrial wall, a collection of fluid is seen. Inferior to the right atrium, the aorta (AO) is seen, with dashes corresponding to aortic leaflet closure during diastole (220 bpm).

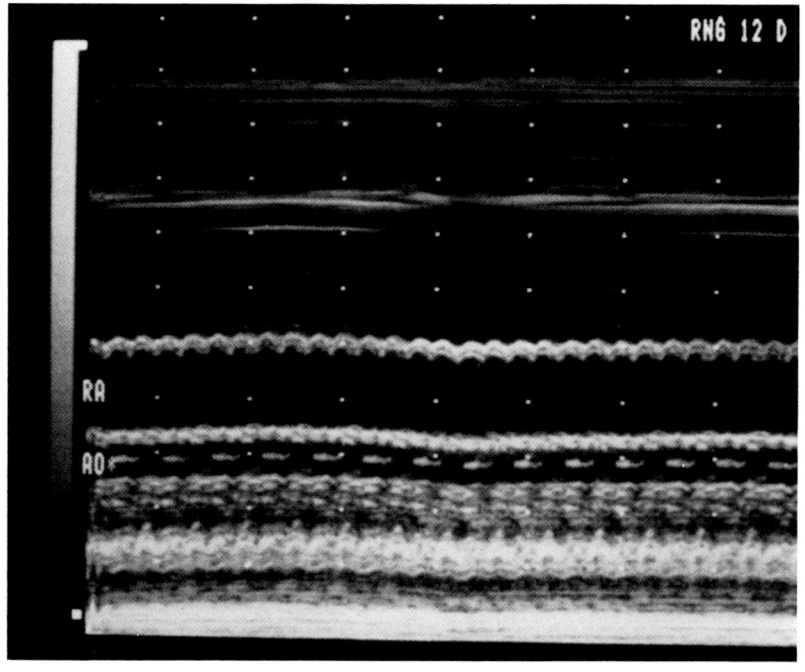

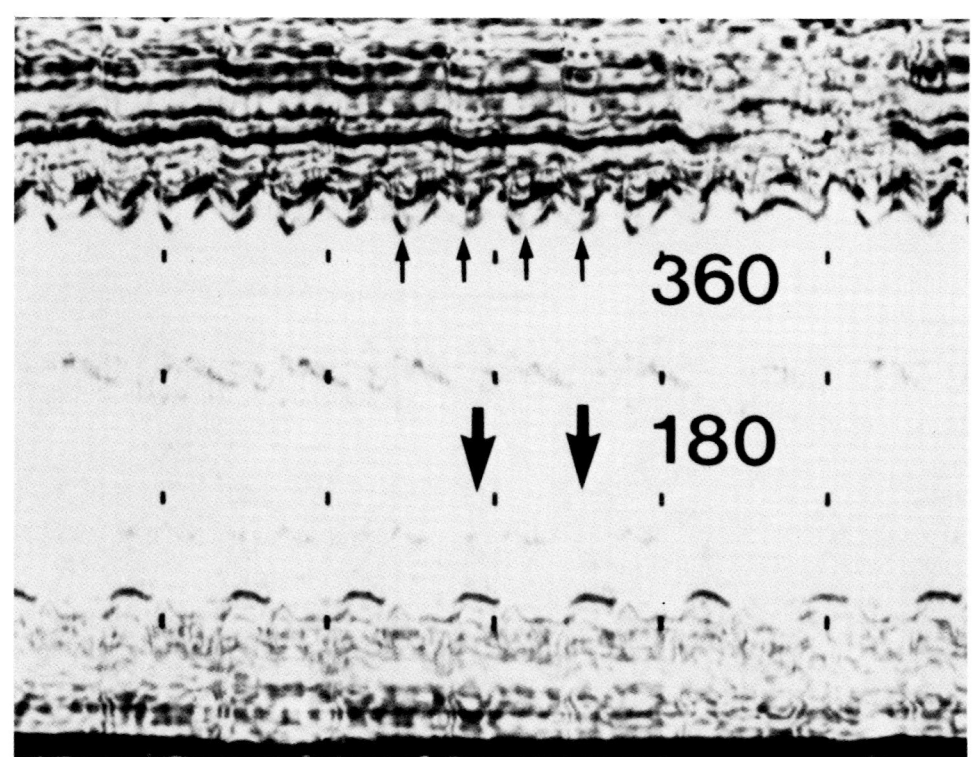

Fig. 7–12. M-mode echocardiogram from a fetus with atrial flutter (atrial rate 360 bpm) with 2:1 block (ventricular rate 180 bpm). The fetal monitoring strip from this fetus is shown in Figure 7–2.

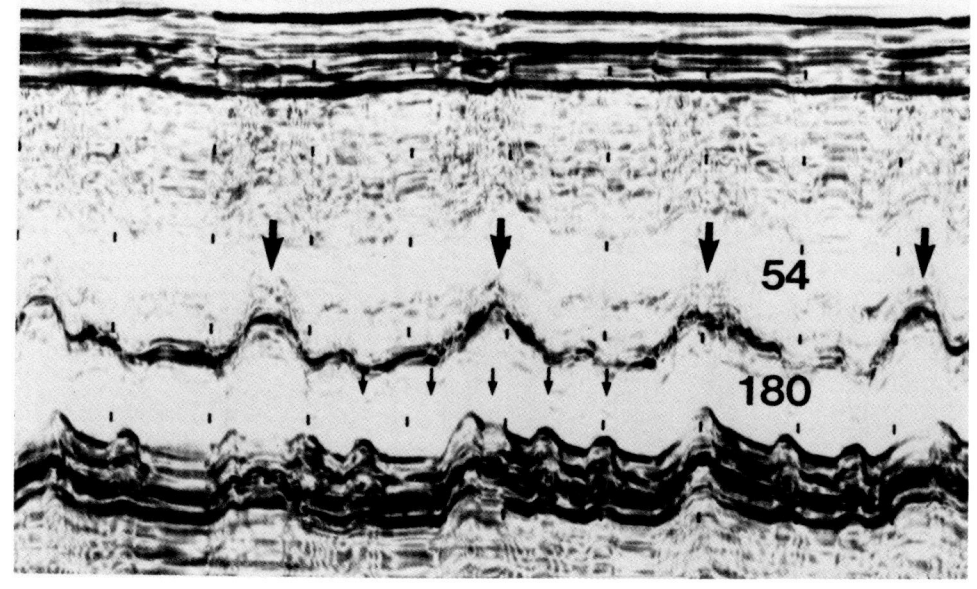

Fig. 7–13. M-mode echocardiogram from a fetus with complete heart block. Atrial rate (small arrows) 180 bpm; ventricular rate (large arrows) 54 bpm. The mother, who was asymptomatic, was found to be ANA negative and anti-Ro antibody positive after fetal heart block was diagnosed. The fetus was delivered vaginally at term and had a pacemaker placed after 48 hours.

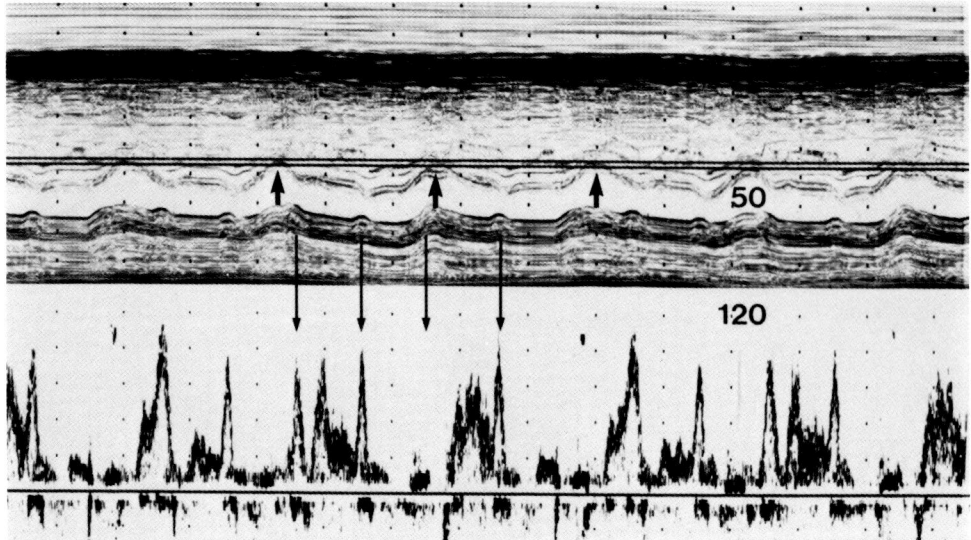

Fig. 7–14. M-mode and Doppler flow velocity tracing across the tricuspid valve of a fetus with congenital heart block. Large arrows: tricuspid valve motion during systole (ventricular wall motion at 50 bpm); small arrows: atrial wall motion and simultaneous flow into the right ventricle with atrial contraction (120 bpm).

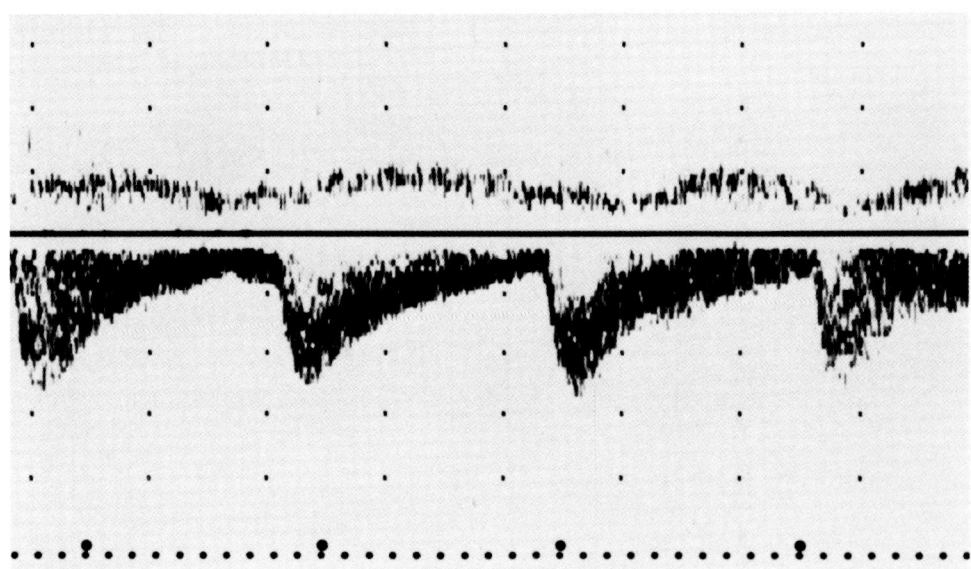

Fig. 7–15. Doppler flow velocity tracing from the umbilical artery and vein of a fetus with congenital heart block. Note the decrease in diastolic velocities due to the long duration between contractions. Fluctuations are also seen in the umbilical vein tracing. Large dots are 1 second apart.

REFERENCES

1. Shenker L: Fetal cardiac arrhythmias. Obstet Gynecol Surv 34:561–572, 1979.
2. Reed KL, Sahn DJ, Marx GR, et al: Cardiac Doppler flows during fetal arrhythmias: Physiologic consequences. Obstet Gynecol 70:1–6, 1987.
3. Kleinman CS, Copel JA, Weinstein EM, et al: In utero diagnosis and treatment of fetal supraventricular tachycardia. Semin Perinatol 9:113–129, 1985.
4. Shenker L, Reed KL, Anderson CF, et al: Congenital heart block and cardiac anomalies in the absence of maternal connective tissue disease. Am J Obstet Gynecol 157:248–253, 1987.

8

Color Flow Mapping
By David J. Sahn

It is obvious, when one looks at the 3.5- or 5-MHz color flow mapping images of fetuses, that some of the problems of lateral resolution related to ultrasound imaging of the heart of the unborn fetus are intensified in color flow mapping in a fashion that allows flow to spread beyond the confines of where it really is. In other words, neither the resolution capabilities nor the flow mapping rasters for the selective analysis of flow in an area at depth from the skin nor the spatial or temporal resolution of flow mapping have been optimized for the evaluation of the fetal cardiovascular system [1,2].

Of substantial importance to contributions of flow mapping will be selective gating modes that allow the specific analysis of a small area within the two-dimensional image at some depth from the transducer. This will necessitate a high-density number of gates, packed axially and radially, with selectable angulation from the transducer. Appropriate magnification modes will be required to enhance the area and bring up low-velocity flow from poor signal-to-noise areas through dynamic range adjustments. These modes should improve, rather than degrade, the image during magnification. Redisplay and remapping of digitally recorded cine loops to bring out detail are also going to be of substantial import in recording and reviewing the information. Nonetheless, even with present day and evolving color flow mapping systems, there are substantial utilities for fetal color flow mapping, which will be illustrated by the selected observations defined in the examples to follow.

The first classification of observations helped by flow mapping is in the definition of vascular channels and the shape of chambers that may not be clearly defined by the echo information, either because of its resolution or because of muscle bundles, irregular intrusions on the lumen, or confusing shadows or echo free spaces.

The second type of benefit is in defining the relationship between tissue and structure as it relates to communications (that is, telling *real* holes from artificial holes, for instance, defining the true diameter of the foramen ovale or clearly defining unequivocally the presence of a ventricular septal defect).

The last category of observations relate to proper implementation of the spectral variance algorithm, which produces the characteristic mosaic on a color flow map to define turbulent flow. This display quickly draws the eye to areas of the circulation that are abnormal aiding in shortening examination time and producing more specific semi-quantitative observations.

This chapter was prepared by David J. Sahn, M.D., F.A.C.C., Division of Pediatric Cardiology, University of California, San Diego.

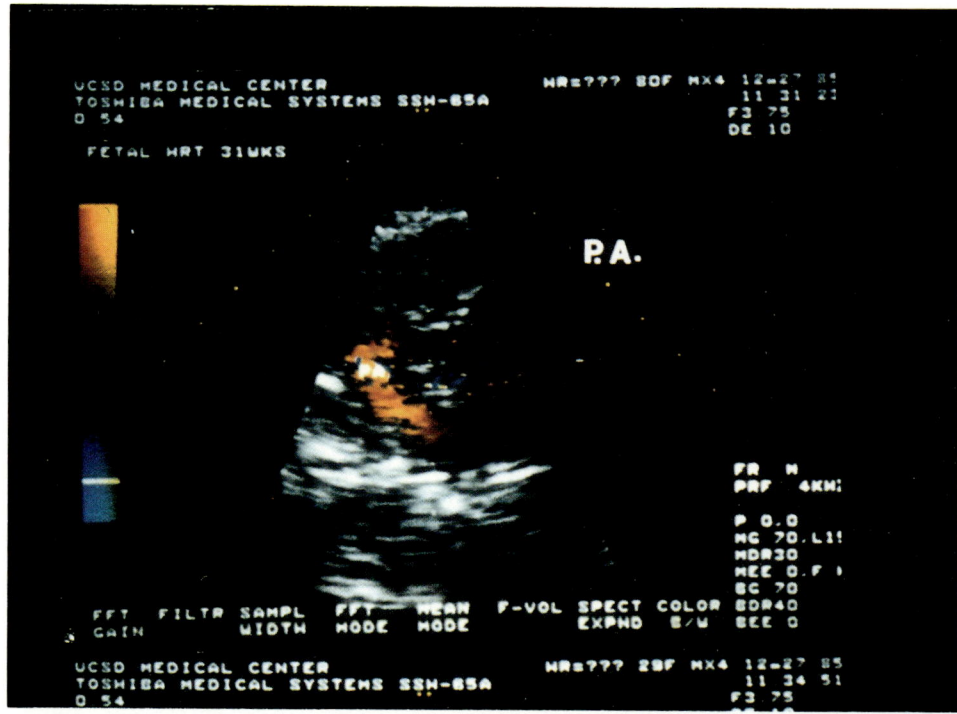

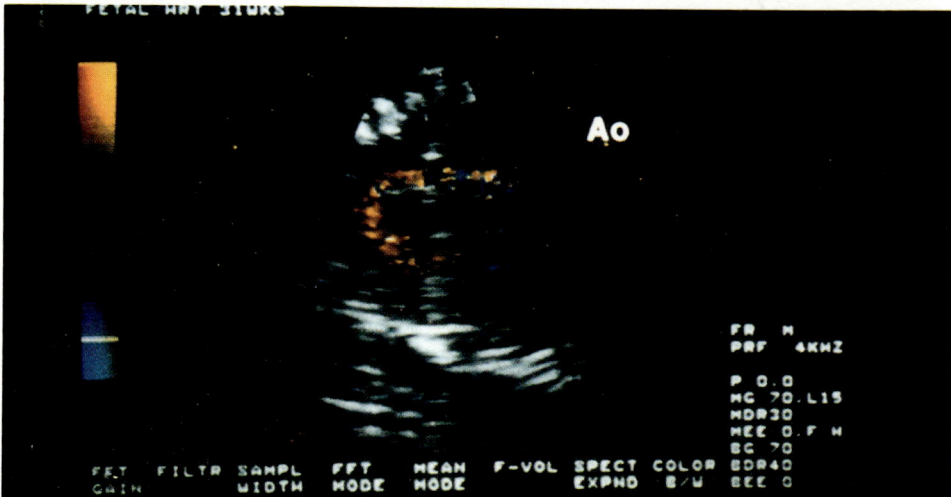

Fig. 8-1. Color flow mapping of the pulmonary artery (PA) and aortic arch (AO) in a 31-week fetus.

CATEGORY I: THE SHAPE OF VESSELS AND CHAMBERS

As can be seen from Figure 8-1, the aortic arch and/or the pulmonary artery and its curvature can easily be defined from the color flow map. The color flow map defines the tight curvature of the aortic arch and the

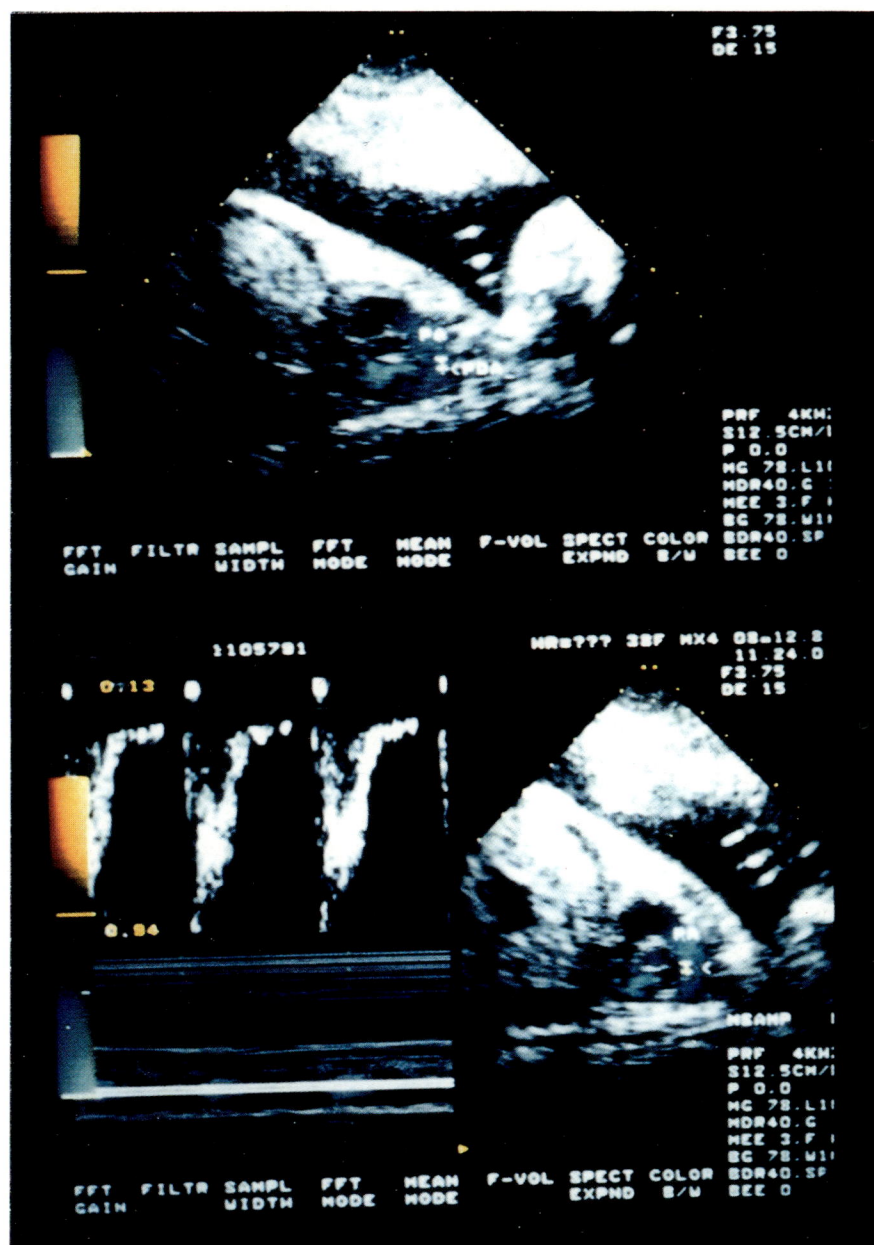

Fig. 8-2. Color flow mapping of the fetal pulmonary artery. PA = pulmonary artery; PDA = patent ductus arteriosus.

gradual tapering of the aortic arch. This enhances tissue identification of the arch of the aorta, which is sometimes difficult due to the intrusion of reverberations and artifacts on what should be the clean lumen. Our observations suggested that normal tapering of the aortic arch is different and clearly definable as abnormal in the fetus at risk for coarctation [3].

Figure 8-2 defines the more distal end of the pulmonary outflow tract near its insertion into the aorta, showing the narrowest area in that

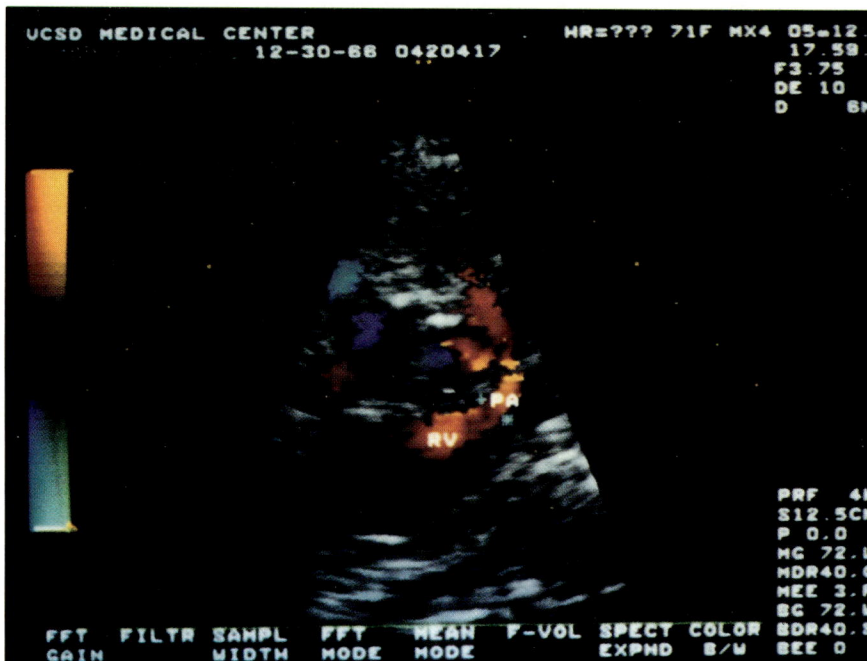

Fig. 8–3. Color flow mapping of the distal right ventricular outflow tract in a fetus with infundibular obstruction in a complex case of transposition of the great arteries. PA=pulmonary artery; RV=right ventricle.

channel as the lumen of the ductus arteriosus. Elegant work has been done by Huhta [4]; it suggests that the diagnosis of ductal constriction can, in fact, be made.

Figure 8–3 shows an example of a complex case of transposition. The flow map defined an area of infundibular obstruction in the distal right ventricular outflow tract that bore extremely close resemblance to the angiogram. The hypoplasia of the pulmonary valve area, with good-sized pulmonary arteries, had been noticed, but the infundibular and long, tubular obstruction of the outflow tract was much more evident on the color flow map.

In Figure 8–4 anatomy suggestive of tetralogy of Fallot, large cystic areas, were visualized within the lungs. The color flow map was quite helpful in defining these as areas containing flow, substantiating a diagnosis of tetralogy with absent pulmonary valve. The to-and-fro flow pattern across the right ventricular outflow tract was helpful in that regard (although not illustrated).

CATEGORY II: INTERCIRCULATORY COMMUNICATIONS

The second type of observations define intercirculatory communications and allow discrimination of true dropout from false septal defects. In Figure

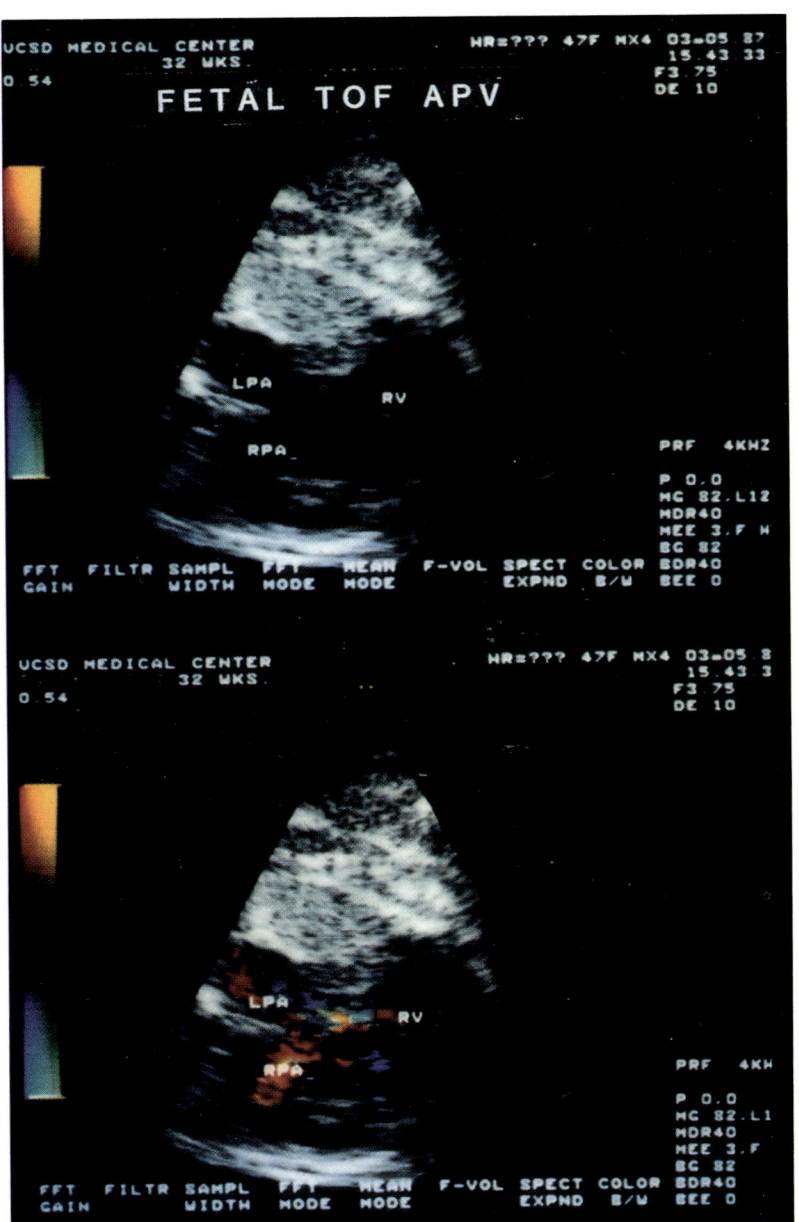

Fig. 8–4. Color flow mapping of dilated areas with flow in the fetal chest in a case of tetralogy of Fallot with absent pulmonary valve (APV). The dilated areas are right (RPA) and left (LPA) pulmonary arteries. RV = right ventricle.

8–5, also from the patient shown on Figure 8–4, the tetralogy with absent pulmonary valve, the ventricular septal defect is visualized in the subaortic area and can be seen shunting right to left. The flow away from the transducer is seen clearly, along with some associate turbulence in the aorta. The abnormal pulmonary artery dynamics, with no ductus arteriosus, limited all flow from the right ventricle to the back-and-forth flow in the right ventricular outflow tract or to a right-to-left shunt across the ventricular septal defect both in systole and diastole.

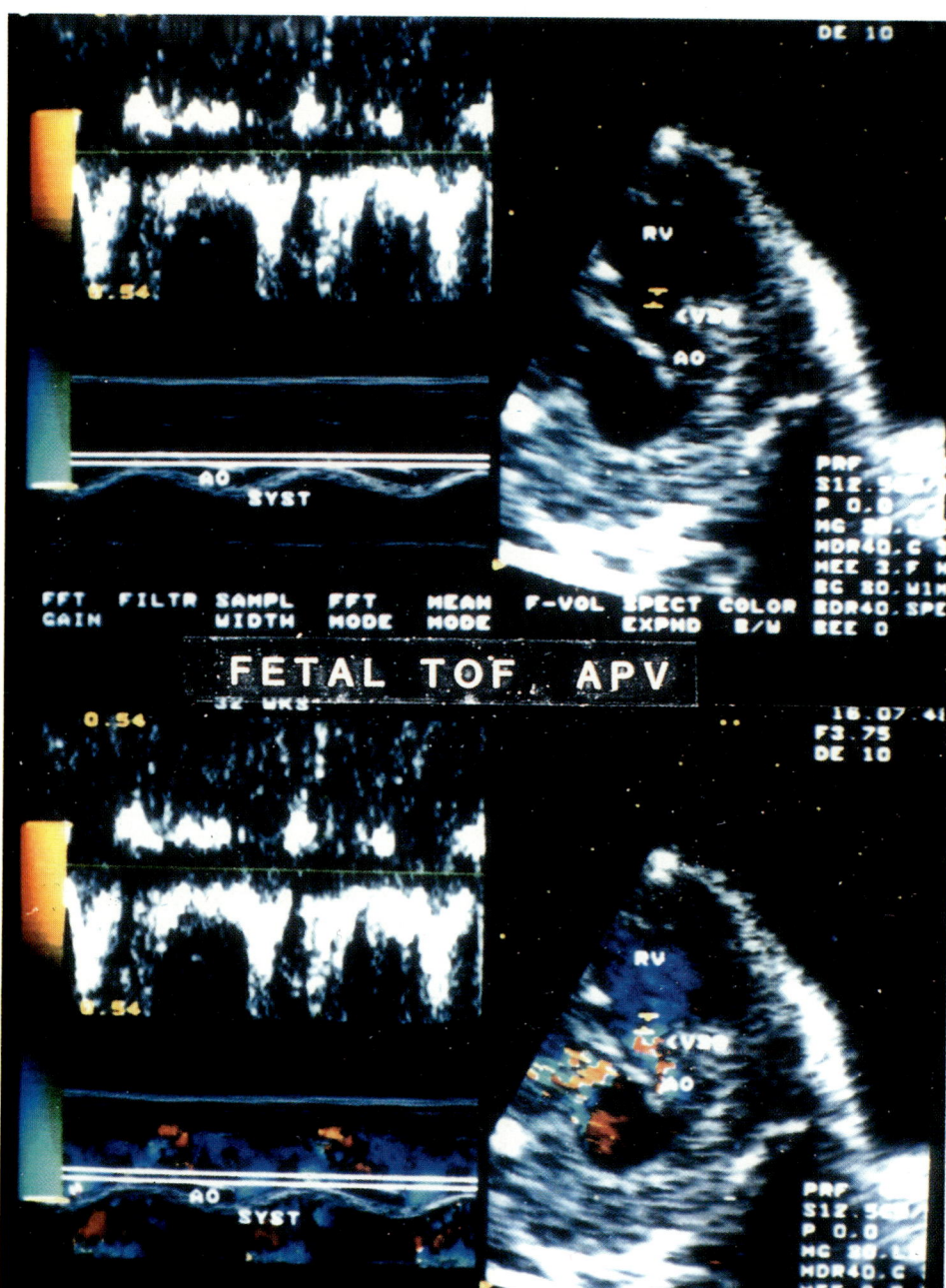

Fig. 8–5. Color flow mapping of the ventricular septal defect (VSD) from the case in Figure 8–4 with tetralogy of Fallot (TOF) with absent pulmonary valve (APV). RV= right ventricle; AO=aorta; Syst=systole.

Figure 8–6 is an illustration in the color flow map, with the flow approaching the transducer, across what looks like the membranous septum. This is a low velocity, minimally aliased shunt, as shown on the QM mode on the lower left with a late systolic and diastolic component. The passage of flow clearly crossing an area of septal dropout allowed waveform interrogation showing a pattern easily distinguishable from atrioventricular valve flow. The latter would be going away from the transducer in this view. The flow map aids in characterizing a low-velocity left-to-right shunt through a ventricular septal defect (a much more characteristic pattern in isolated ventricular septal defects).

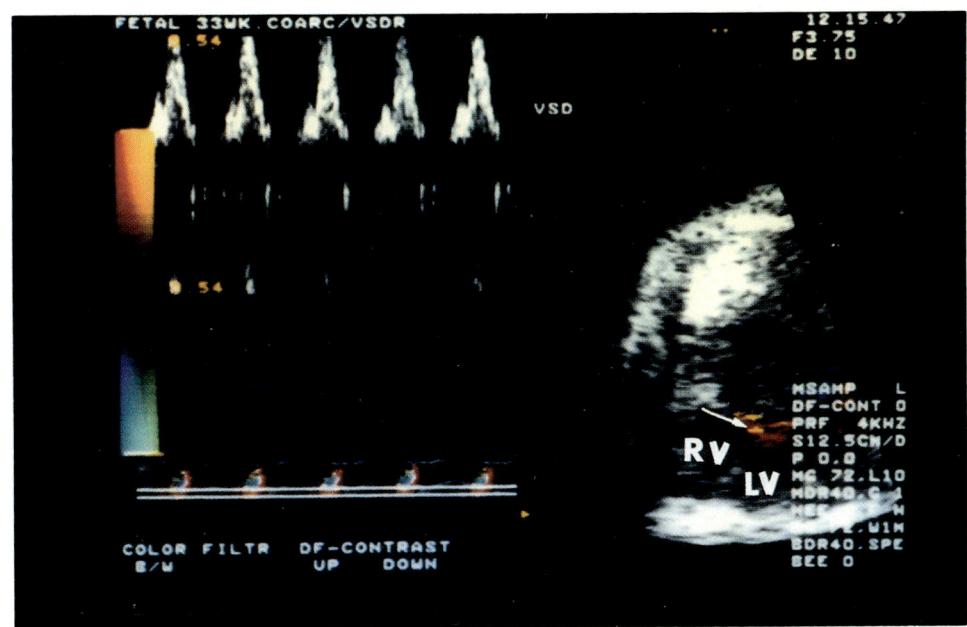

Fig. 8-6. Color flow mapping in a fetus with a ventricular septal defect (VSD). RV = right ventricle; LV = left ventricle.

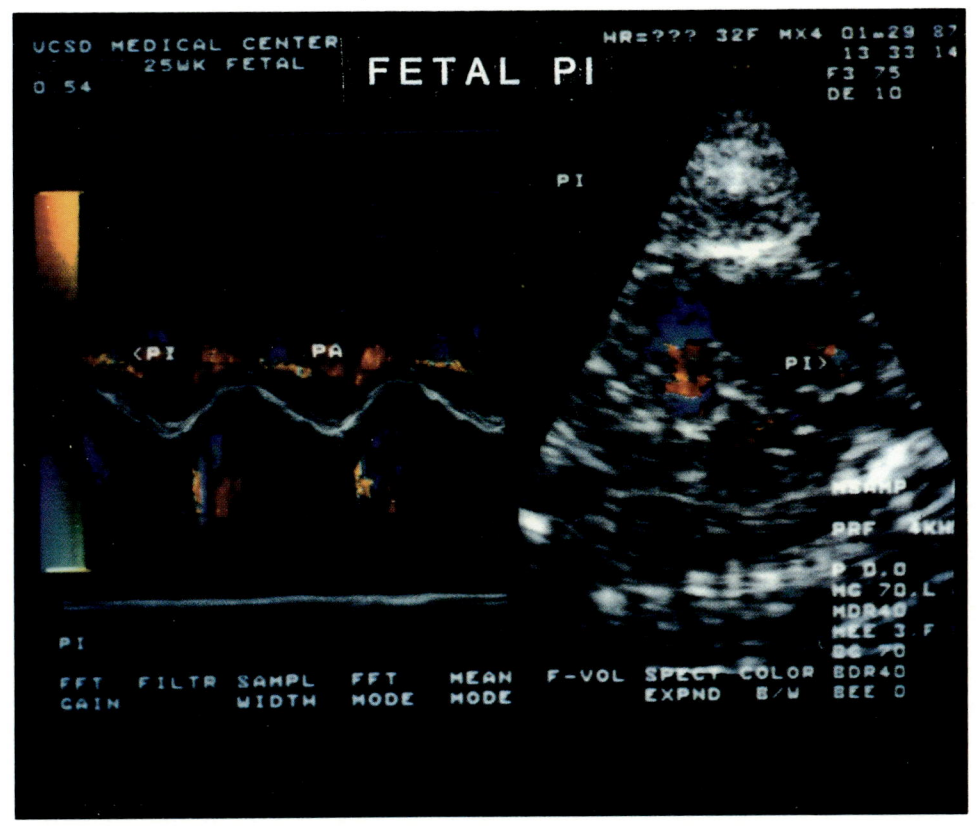

Fig. 8-7. Color flow mapping of a fetus with pulmonary insufficiency (PI). PA = pulmonary artery.

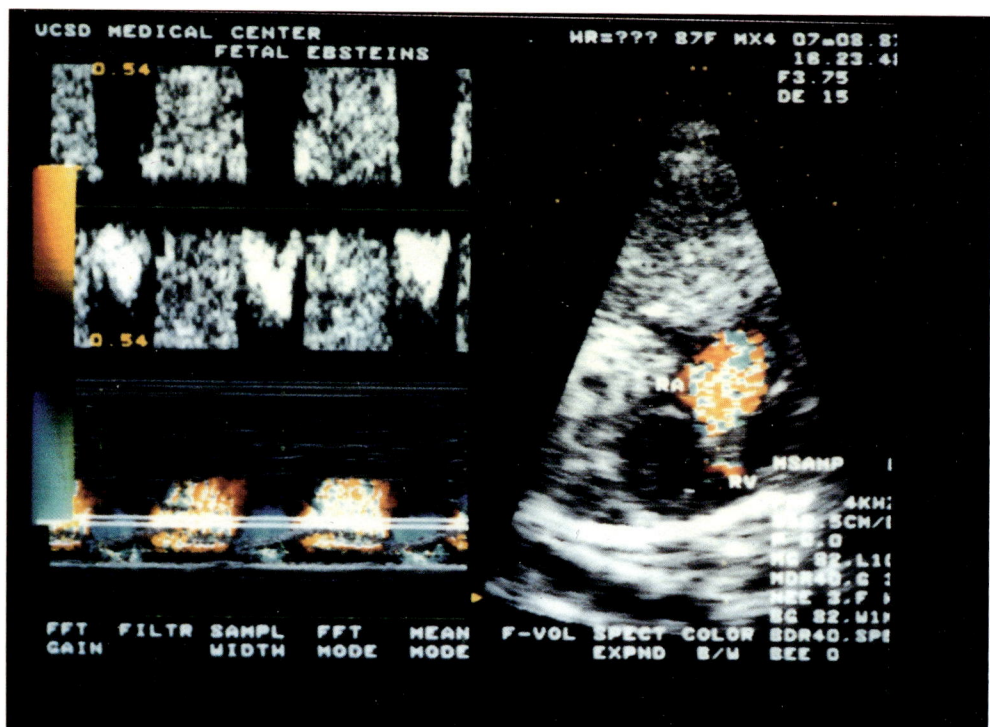

Fig. 8–8. Color flow mapping of a fetus with Ebstein's anomaly. RA=right atrium; RV=right ventricle.

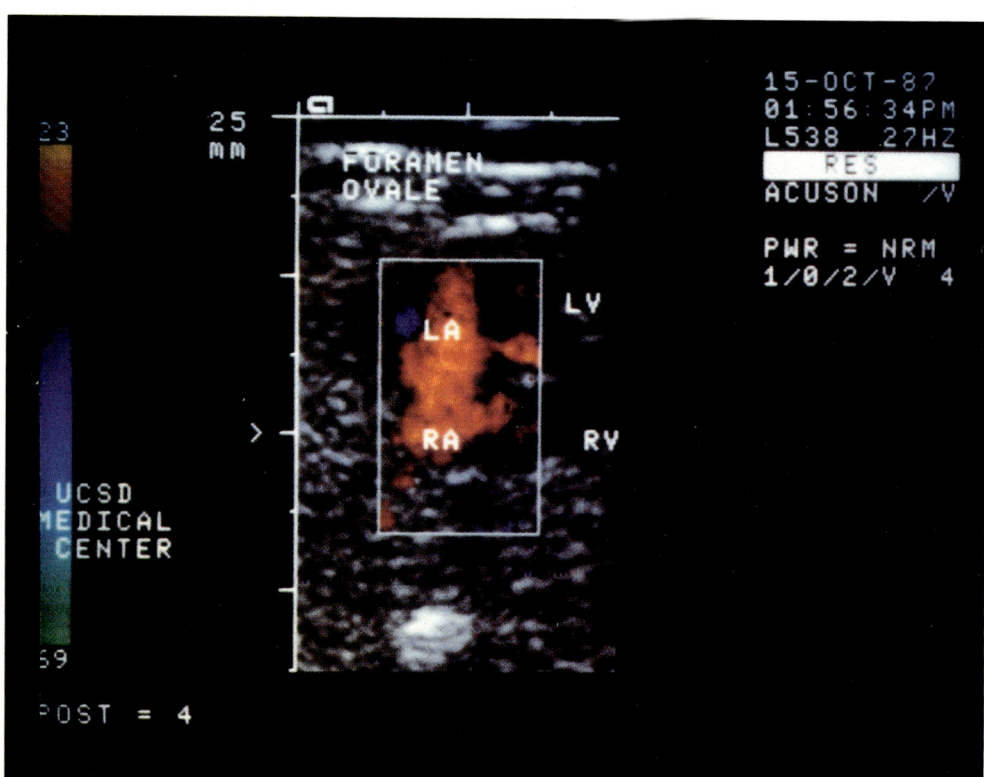

Fig. 8–9. Color flow mapping of the fetal foramen ovale. LA = left atrium; RA = right atrium; LV = left ventricle; RV = right ventricle.

CATEGORY III: VARIANT "TURBULENT" FLOW

The third class of observations are those involving the variance display. Figure 8–7 shows a fetus with documented ductal constriction in whom an abnormal flow pattern was observed. This figure documents reverse flow at the level of the pulmonary valve, proving the presence of pulmonary insufficiency in the unborn fetus who also had tricuspid insufficiency. The characteristic flow returning toward the transducer through the pulmonary valve was visualized on the color flow image. A mosaic pattern of variance can be seen on the QM mode to represent early diastolic pulmonary insufficiency. Note the color flow map image has a combination of mosaic colors, which suggests disorganized flow.

A more graphic example is shown in Figure 8–8, which shows a patient with prenatal diagnosis of Ebstein's malformation, first made at 28 weeks gestation. The tricuspid valve is displaced into the right ventricle. The accelerating flow coming toward the transducer shows a signal alias from red to blue proximal to the tricuspid valve in the right ventricular cavity. The flow then erupts into the right atrium as a highly turbulent spray. It can also be seen on the QM mode and shows multiple aliases on the sampled spectral Doppler ultrasound image, documenting wide open tricuspid insufficiency in a fetus who subsequently was stillborn.

Figure 8–9 shows the early results of an ultrasound system that has been more adequately optimized for fetal sampling. In this example, a magnification mode has been employed with a localized area of flow mapping to define a high-density flow data matrix in the atrial cavity; the dynamic range has been adjusted to bring up the color intensity of what is a relatively low-velocity right atrial to left atrial foramen ovale shunt. This defines the diameter of the foramen jet flow to be about 4 mm, a normal size for foramenal flow for a 19-week fetus; the foramen is usually two-thirds the size of the aortic root.

Only through more optimized sampling, with higher resolution systems, will truly adequate results for the application of fetal color flow technologies be forthcoming.

REFERENCES

1. Kasai C, Namekawa K: In Omoto R (ed): A Color Atlas of Real-time Two-Dimensional Echocardiography, Ed. 2. Tokyo: Shindan-To-Chiryo Co., 1987.
2. Sahn DJ: Real-time two-dimensional echocardiographic Doppler flow mapping. Circulation 71:849–853, 1985.
3. Hornberger LK, Pesonen E, Simpson IA, Hagen-Ansert S, Sahn DJ: Echocardiographic study of the morphology and growth of the aortic arch in the human fetus: Observations related to the prenatal diagnosis of coarctation (abstr). J Am Coll Cardiol 11:10, 1988.
4. Huhta JC, Moise KJ, Fisher DJ, Sharif DS, Wasserstrum N, Martin C: Detection and quantitation of constriction of the fetal ductus arteriosus by Doppler echocardiography. Circulation 75:406–412, 1987.

INDEX

Anti-Ro antibody, 1, 3, 90–91, 106, 118, 123–124
  association with complete heart block, 1, 90–91
Aorta, 18–19, 21–25, 28, 30, 34–41, 43–45, 104–106, 120, 122
  ascending, 6, 9, 13, 18–19, 21–25, 28, 30–31, 37, 103
  coarctation of the, 12, 30, 37, 71, 80
  descending, 5, 8–9, 13, 20–21, 25, 31, 34–41
    Doppler echocardiography, 109–110
  interruption of the arch, 71, 78–79
Aortic arch, 13, 20–21, 25, 28–30, 37–43, 71, 75, 78–80
  color flow mapping of, 126
  interruption of, 71, 78–79
Aortic valve, 2, 13, 22–25, 30, 41, 43, 109–111, 113, 122
  atresia, 25, 30, 47, 52
  atrial flutter, 106
  Doppler velocities, 109–111, 113, 122
    volume flow calculations, 111
  size, 21, 30–31, 43, 103–104
  stenosis, 25
Arch
  aortic, 13, 20–21, 25, 28–30, 37–43, 71, 75, 78–80
    color flow mapping, 126
  pulmonary artery/ductus, 13, 20–21, 30, 37, 41–43
Arrhythmias, 1–2, 43, 103–107, 115–124
  atrial bigeminy, 122
  atrial flutter, 104, 106, 115, 117–118, 122–123
    fetal heart rate monitoring, 117
    M-mode echocardiography, 104, 106, 117, 122–123
  complete heart block, 103–104, 106, 115, 118, 123–124
    association with anti-Ro antibody, 1, 90–91, 106, 118, 123–124
    association with atrioventricular canal defect, 67, 69, 81
    association with great vessel abnormalities, 89–91
    Doppler echocardiography, 124
    M-mode echocardiography, 103–104, 106, 123–124
    and heart failure, 83, 118
  premature atrial contractions, 103–105, 115–116, 118–120
    Doppler echocardiography, 118–120
    M-mode echocardiography, 103–105, 116, 120
  premature ventricular contractions, 103–104, 115, 118, 121
    Doppler echocardiography, 118, 121
    M-mode echocardiography, 103–104, 121
  supraventricular tachycardia, 83, 86–87, 104, 115, 118, 122
    M-mode echocardiography, 83, 87, 104, 122
Atrial bigeminy, 122
Atrial contraction, premature. *See* Premature atrial contractions
Atrial flutter, 104, 106, 115, 117–118, 122–123
  fetal heart rate monitoring, 117
  M-mode echocardiography, 104, 106, 122–123
Atrial septal defect, 2–3, 12, 67, 68, 70, 76, 95
  see also Atrioventricular canal defect
Atrioventricular canal defect, 2, 12, 67, 69–70, 81, 112–113
  association with complete heart block, 67, 69, 81
  association with Down syndrome, 2, 67, 70
  Doppler flow velocities, 112–113
Atrium, 5–9, 12–19, 21–28, 30–31, 38–41, 43–45, 103, 105–106, 115–116, 118, 121–122
  common, 69
  right, enlarged, 59–61, 67, 83, 86–87, 118

Bigeminy, atrial, 122
Blood flow
  color mapping, 125–133
  velocity, 110–111
Blood pressure, 8

Cardiomyopathy, 12
Cerebral vessels
　Doppler echocardiography, 109–111
Chromosomes, abnormal, as an indication for fetal echocardiography, 1, 71
　associated cardiac anomalies, 2–3, 64, 71
Circulation, fetal, 5–9
Coarctation of the aorta, 12, 30, 37, 71, 80
Color flow mapping, 114, 125–133
Complete heart block, 103–104, 106, 115, 118, 123–124
　association with anti-Ro antibody, 1, 3, 90–91, 106, 118, 123–124
　association with atrioventricular canal defect, 67, 69, 81
　association with great vessel abnormalities, 89–91
　Doppler echocardiography, 124
　M-mode echocardiography, 103–104, 106, 123–124
Compliance, ventricular, 8–9
　and Doppler examinations, 111
Congenital lobar emphysema, 89, 96
Connective tissue disease, 1
Cystic adenomatoid malformation of the lung, 89, 96

Dextrocardia, 2, 11, 12
Diabetes, 1–2, 65, 83, 85, 105–106, 107
Diaphragmatic hernia, 68, 89, 95
Doppler echocardiography, 9, 43, 109–114, 118–121, 124
　aortic, 109–111, 113
　in arrhythmias, 118–121, 124
　cerebral vessels, 109–111
　descending aorta, 109–111
　and Frank-Starling mechanism, 111
　in hypoplastic left heart syndrome, 112–113
　in hypertensive pregnancies, 112
　inferior vena cava, 109, 111
　in intrauterine growth retardation, 111–112
　maternal arteries, 109–111
　mitral valve, 109–111, 113
　normal fetal values, 110–111
　and post-extrasystolic potentiation, 111
　pulmonary artery, 109–111, 113
　tricuspid valve, 109–111, 113, 119, 124
　in twin–twin transfusion, 98–99
　umbilical artery, 109–112, 124
　umbilical vein, 109–111, 124
　and ventricular compliance, 111
　volume flow calculations, 109–111
Double-outlet right heart, 12, 25, 65, 71, 76, 112–113
　Doppler echocardiography, 112–113

Down syndrome
　and atrioventricular canal defect, 2, 67, 70
　Doppler echocardiography, 112
　and tetralogy of Fallot, 2, 71, 72–74
Ductus arteriosus. See Patent ductus arteriosus

Ebstein's anomaly, 2, 12, 52, 62–63, 112–113
　color flow mapping, 132–133
　Doppler echocardiography, 112–113
Ectopia cordis, 12, 89, 97
Effusion
　pericardial, 12, 43, 83, 85, 87, 103–105, 118
　pleural, 67, 83, 86, 106, 118, 122
Endocardial cushion defect. See Atrioventricular canal defect
Endocardial fibroelastosis, 83, 88

Family history, as an indication for fetal echocardiography, 1
Fetal cardiac examinations, indications, 1
Fetal, indications for echocardiography, 1
Five-chamber view, 13, 18–19, 43
Foramen ovale, 2–3, 5, 7, 9, 12–17, 25–27, 47, 67
　color flow mapping, 132–133
Four-chamber view, 12–17, 43
　apical, 12–15
　from the base, 16–17
　long axis, 25–27
Fractional shortening, 25, 103–105

Great vessel views, 21–25, 28–30, 34–43
　long axis, 21–24, 30, 43
　short axis, 30, 34–36, 43
　abnormal, 67, 71–80, 90–91

Heart block. See Complete heart block
Heart rate, 8
Hemoglobin, 8–9
Hydrops, 2, 118
Hypertrophy
　septal, 83, 85, 105–107
　ventricular, 1, 12, 67, 69, 83–85, 105
Hypoplasia, 12
　left ventricle/heart, 12, 47–51
　　Doppler echocardiography, 112–113
　right ventricle/heart, 12, 52–53, 58, 75

Inferior vena cava, 6, 9, 21–24, 30, 43–45, 80, 81
　and left atrial isomerism, 67, 81
Intra-atrial septum, 12–19, 25–27
Intrauterine growth retardation, 2, 83, 89, 104, 112
　Doppler echocardiography, 111–112
Isoimmunization, 1

Isomerism, atrial, 67, 69, 81

Left ventricular outflow tract, 5, 25, 28

Maternal diseases, as an indication for fetal echocardiography, 1
Mitral valve, 12–19, 26–27, 31, 43, 103, 105, 109–111, 113, 116
  atresia, 47, 52
  Doppler velocities, 109–111, 113
    volume flow calculations, 111
  enlarged, 56, 66
  size, 43
M-mode echocardiography, 31, 43, 83, 103–107, 115–118, 120–124
  atrial bigeminy, 122
  atrial flutter, 104, 106, 122–123
  complete heart block, 103–104, 106, 123–124
  fractional shortening, 25, 103–105
  pericardial effusion, 103–105
  pleural effusion, 104, 106, 122
  premature atrial contraction, 103–105, 116, 118
  premature ventricular contraction, 103, 115, 118, 121
  septal hypertrophy, 105, 107
  supraventricular tachycardia, 87, 104, 122
  ventricular hypertrophy, 83, 105

Oxygen, partial pressure of, 8–9
Oxygen saturation, 8–9

Patent ductus arteriosus, 2–3, 5–9, 12–13, 20–21, 25, 29–31, 34–37, 41, 47, 71
  color flow mapping, 127
  constriction, 128
    color flow mapping, 131, 133
  with Ebstein's anomaly, 63
Pericardial effusion, 12, 43, 83, 85, 87, 103–105, 118
Pericardium, 12
Phenylketonuria, 1–2
Pleural effusion, 67, 86, 106, 118, 122
Post-extrasystolic potentiation, 105, 111
Premature atrial contractions, 103–105, 115–116, 118–120
  Doppler echocardiography, 118–120
  M-mode echocardiography, 103–105, 116, 118
Premature ventricular contractions, 103–104, 115, 118, 121
  Doppler echocardiography, 118, 121
  M-mode echocardiography, 103–104, 118, 121
Pulmonary artery, 8, 13, 20–22, 25, 28–31, 34–41, 43–45, 57, 126–127
  color flow mapping, 126–127
  enlarged, 57

Pulmonary valve, 2, 13, 20–25, 29–31, 34–36, 43, 109–111, 113
  atresia, 30, 52, 59–61, 112–113
  Doppler velocities, 109–111, 113
    volume flow calculations, 111
  insufficiency
    color flow mapping, 131
  size, 21, 30–31, 43
  stenosis, 3
    Doppler echocardiography, 112–113
    color flow mapping, 128, 129
    and tetralogy of Fallot, 71
Pulmonary vein, 12–17, 25–27, 29, 44–45, 80
  anomalous, 2–3, 82

Resistance, vascular, 8–9
Rhabdomyoma, 89, 92
Right ventricular outflow tract, 5, 13, 18–25, 29, 31

Septal defects. *See* Atrial septal defect, Ventricular septal defect
Septum
  intra-atrial 12–19, 25–27
  ventricular, 5, 12–19, 25–28, 31
    hypertrophy, 83, 85, 105–107
Short axis/great vessel view, 31, 34–36, 43
Single ventricle, 52, 54–55, 77
Situs inversus, 11, 12, 83, 89, 93–94
Superior vena cava, 8, 14–17, 21–24, 26–30, 43–45
Supraventricular tachycardia, 83, 86–87, 104, 115, 118, 122
  M-mode echocardiography, 83, 87, 104, 122

Tachycardia, supraventricular, 83, 86–87, 104, 115, 118, 122
Teratogens, as an indication for fetal echocardiography, 1
Teratoma, 89
Tetralogy of Fallot, 2, 12, 30, 71–74, 105, 112–113
  Doppler velocities, 112–113
  color flow mapping, 128–130
Thoracopagus, 100
Total anomalous venous return, 80, 82
Transposition of the great vessels, 25, 30, 37, 53, 71, 75
  color flow mapping, 128
Tricuspid valve, 12–19, 21–24, 26–31, 34–36, 43–45, 109–111, 113, 119, 121, 124
  atresia, 12, 52–53, 56–58, 66, 75, 112
  Doppler echocardiography, 113
  Doppler velocities, 109–111, 113, 119, 124
    volume flow calculations, 113

insufficiency, 3, 12, 52, 62, 131, 133, 114, 118
size, 43
Truncus arteriosus, 30, 54, 71, 77
Tumor, 12, 83, 89, 92
Twins, 67, 89, 98–100
  conjoined, 89, 100
Twin–twin transfusion, 89, 98–99

Umbilical artery, 8–9, 101
  Doppler studies, 109–112, 118, 120, 124
Umbilical cord, 89, 101
  three vessel, 101
  two vessel, 64, 101
Umbilical vein, 6, 8–9, 101, 109–111, 124
  Doppler studies, 109–111, 124
Univentricular heart. *See* Single ventricle

Ventricle, 1, 5–9, 12–24, 25–28, 31, 34–37, 41, 43–45, 103–105, 115, 118–119
  double outlet right heart, 12, 25, 65, 71, 76
  hypoplasia, 12
    right, 52, 75
    left, 47–51
  single, 12, 52, 54–55, 77
  volume flow, 8, 105
Ventricular hypertrophy, 1, 12, 65, 83–85, 105
  causes, 83
  with left atrial isomerism and atrioventricular canal defect, 67, 69
Ventricular premature contraction. *See* Premature ventricular contractions
Ventricular septal defect, 2–3, 12, 25, 53, 56, 58, 64–70, 75, 79
  color flow mapping, 129, 130, 131, 133
  with tetralogy of Fallot, 73
Ventricular septum, 5, 12–19, 25–28, 31
  hypertrophy, 83, 85, 105–107
Ventricular short axis view, 31